Instructor's Guide
for

ESSENTIALS OF PSYCHIATRIC MENTAL HEALTH NURSING
2nd Edition

Mary C. Townsend, RN, MN, CS

Clinical Nurse Specialist
Adult Psychiatric/Mental Health Nursing
Counseling Center of Southeast Oklahoma
Antlers, Oklahoma

Former Assistant Professor and
Coordinator, Mental Health Nursing
Kramer School of Nursing
Oklahoma City University
Oklahoma City, Oklahoma

F. A. Davis Company
1915 Arch Street
Philadelphia, PA 19103
www.fadavis.com

ISBN: 8036-0921-3

Printed in the United States of America

Last digit indicates print number: 10 9 8 7 6 5 4 3 2

As new scientific information becomes available through basic and clinical research, recommended treatments and drug therapies undergo changes. The author(s) and publisher have done everything possible to make this book accurate, up to date, and in accord with accepted standards at the time of publication. The author(s), editors, and publisher are not responsible for errors or omissions or for consequences from application of the book, and make no warranty, expressed or implied, in regard to the contents of the book. Any practice described in this book should be applied by the reader in accordance with professional standards of care used in regard to the unique circumstances that may apply in each situation. The reader is advised always to check product information (package inserts) for changes and new information regarding dose and contraindications before administering any drug. Caution is especially urged when using new or infrequently ordered drugs.

Contents

CHAPTER 1. MENTAL HEALTH AND MENTAL ILLNESS

CHAPTER FOCUS

This chapter focuses on the differentiation between mental health and mental illness. Physical and psychological responses to stress are discussed and cultural influences are explored.

LEARNING OBJECTIVES

After reading this chapter, the student will be able to:
1. Define *mental health* and *mental illness*.
2. Discuss cultural elements that influence attitudes toward mental health and mental illness.
3. Identify physiological responses to stress.
4. Discuss concepts of anxiety and grief as psychological responses to stress.
5. Describe the *DSM-IV-TR* multiaxial evaluation system for classification of mental disorders.

KEY TERMS

fight-or-flight syndrome
ego defense mechanisms
anxiety
grief
neurosis
psychosis
anticipatory grieving
bereavement overload
Diagnostic and Statistical Manual of Mental Disorders, 4th ed, Text Revision (DSM-IV-TR)

CHAPTER OUTLINE/LECTURE NOTES

I. Introduction
   A. The concepts of mental health and mental illness are culturally defined.
   B. Individuals experience both physical and psychological responses to stress.
II. Mental Health
   A. Defined as: "The successful adaptation to stressors from the internal or external environment, evidenced by thoughts, feelings, and behaviors that are age-appropriate and congruent with local and cultural norms."
III. Mental Illness

A. Defined as: "Maladaptive responses to stressors from the internal or external environment, evidenced by thoughts, feelings, and behaviors that are incongruent with the local and cultural norms and interfere with the individual's social, occupational, and/or physical functioning."

B. Horwitz describes cultural influences that affect how individuals view mental illness. These include *incomprehensibility* (the inability of the general population to understand the motivation behind the behavior) and *cultural relativity* (the "normality" of behavior is determined by the culture).

IV. Physical and Psychological Responses to Stress

A. Physical responses

1. Hans Selye defined stress as "the state manifested by a specific syndrome which consists of all the nonspecifically induced changes within a biological system." This syndrome of physical symptoms has come to be known as the **fight-or-flight syndrome**.

2. Selye called this general reaction of the body to stress the *general adaptation syndrome (GAS)*. He described the reaction in three distinct stages.

   a. Alarm reaction stage. During this stage, the physiological responses of the fight-or-flight syndrome are initiated.

   b. Stage of resistance. The individual uses the physiological responses of the first stage as a defense in the attempt to adapt to the stressor. If adaptation occurs, the third stage is prevented or delayed. Physiological symptoms may disappear.

   c. Stage of exhaustion. Occurs when there is a prolonged exposure to the stressor to which the body has become adjusted. The adaptive energy is depleted, and the individual can no longer draw from the resources for adaptation described in the first two stages. Diseases of adaptation may occur, and, without intervention for reversal, exhaustion and even death ensues.

3. The immediate response. The hypothalamus stimulates the sympathetic nervous system, which results in the following physical effects:

   a. The adrenal medulla releases norepinephrine and epinephrine into the bloodstream.

   b. The pupils of the eye dilate.

   c. Secretion from the lacrimal (tear) glands is increased.

   d. In the lungs, the bronchioles dilate, and the respiration rate is increased.

   e. The force of cardiac contraction increases, as does cardiac output, heart rate, and blood pressure.

   f. GI motility and secretions decrease, and sphincters contract.

   g. In the liver, there is increased glycogenolysis and gluconeogenesis, and a decrease in glycogen synthesis.

   h. The bladder muscle contracts and the sphincter relaxes; there is increased ureter motility.

   i. Secretion from the sweat glands is increased.

   j. Lipolysis occurs in the fat cells.

4. The sustained response. When an individual experiences stress over a long

period of time, the hypothalamus stimulates the pituitary gland to release hormones that produce the following effects:

    a. Adrenocorticotropic hormone (ACTH) stimulates the adrenal cortex to release glucocorticoids and mineralocorticoids, resulting in increased gluconeogenesis and retention of sodium and water and decreased immune and inflammatory responses.

    b. Vasopressin (antidiuretic hormone [ADH]) increases blood pressure through constriction of blood vessels and also increases fluid retention.

    c. Growth hormone has a direct effect on protein, carbohydrate, and lipid metabolism, resulting in increased serum glucose and free fatty acids.

    d. Thyrotropic hormone stimulates the thyroid gland to increase the basal metabolic rate (BMR).

    e. Gonadotropins cause a decrease in secretion of sex hormones resulting in decreased libido and impotence.

  5. It is this chronic response that maintains the body in the aroused condition for extended periods of time that promotes susceptibility to diseases of adaptation.

B. Psychological responses

  1. **Anxiety** and **grief** have been described as two major, primary psychological response patterns to stress. A variety of thoughts, feelings, and behaviors are associated with each of these response patterns. Adaptation is determined by the degree to which the thoughts, feelings, and behaviors interfere with an individual's functioning.

  2. Anxiety

    a. Defined: A diffuse apprehension that is vague in nature and is associated with feelings of uncertainty and helplessness.

    b. Anxiety is extremely common in our society. Mild anxiety is adaptive and can provide motivation for survival.

    c. Peplau identified four levels of anxiety.

      (1) Mild: Seldom a problem. Associated with the tension of day-to-day living. Senses are sharp, motivation is increased, and awareness of the environment is heightened. Learning is enhanced.

      (2) Moderate: Perceptual field diminishes. Less alert to environmental stimuli. Attention span and ability to concentrate decrease, although some learning can still occur. Muscular tension and restlessness may be evident.

      (3) Severe: Perceptual field is so diminished that concentration centers on one detail only or on many extraneous details. Very limited attention span. Physical symptoms may be evident. Virtually all behavior is aimed at relieving the anxiety.

      (4) Panic: The most intense state. Individual is unable to focus on even one detail. Misperceptions of the environment are common, and there may be a loss of contact with reality. Behavior may be characterized by wild and desperate actions or by extreme withdrawal. Human function and communication with others are ineffective. Prolonged

panic anxiety can lead to physical and emotional exhaustion and can be a life-threatening situation

d. Behavioral adaptation responses to anxiety

(1) At the mild level, individuals employ various coping mechanisms to deal with stress. A few of these include eating, drinking, sleeping, physical exercise, smoking, crying, laughing, and talking to someone with whom they feel comfortable.

(2) At the mild to moderate level, **ego defense mechanisms** are called on for protection, such as:

(a) compensation—covering up a real or perceived weakness by emphasizing a trait one considers more desirable.

(b) denial—refusal to acknowledge the existence of a real situation or the feelings associated with it.

(c) displacement—feelings are transferred from one target to another that is considered less threatening or neutral.

(d) identification—an attempt to increase self-worth by acquiring certain attributes and characteristics of an individual one admires.

(e) intellectualization—an attempt to avoid expressing actual emotions associated with a stressful situation by using the intellectual processes of logic, reasoning, and analysis.

(f) introjection—the beliefs and values of another individual are internalized and symbolically become a part of the self, to the extent that the feeling of separateness or distinctness is lost.

(g) isolation—the separation of a thought or a memory from the feeling, tone, or emotions associated with it.

(h) projection—feelings or impulses unacceptable to one's self are attributed to another person.

(i) rationalization—attempting to make excuses or formulate logical reasons to justify unacceptable feelings or behaviors.

(j) reaction formation—preventing unacceptable or undesirable thoughts or behaviors from being expressed by exaggerating opposite thoughts or types of behaviors.

(k) regression—a retreat to an earlier level of development and the comfort measures associated with that level of functioning.

(l) repression—the involuntary blocking of unpleasant feelings and experiences from one's awareness.

(m) sublimation—the rechanneling of drives or impulses that are personally or socially unacceptable into activities that are more tolerable and constructive.

(n) suppression—the voluntary blocking of unpleasant feelings and experiences from one's awareness.

(o) undoing—a mechanism that is used to symbolically negate or cancel out a previous action or experience that one finds intolerable.

(3) Anxiety at the moderate to severe level that remains unresolved over

an extended period of time can contribute to a number of physiological disorders. These may include, but are not limited to, tension and migraine headaches, angina pectoris, obesity, anorexia nervosa, bulimia nervosa, rheumatoid arthritis, ulcerative colitis, gastric and duodenal ulcers, asthma, irritable bowel syndrome, nausea and vomiting, gastritis, cardiac arrhythmias, premenstrual syndrome, muscle spasms, sexual dysfunction, and cancer (discussed in Chapter 17).

(4) Extended periods of repressed severe anxiety can result in psychoneurotic patterns of behaving. Neuroses are psychiatric disturbances characterized by excessive anxiety or depression, disrupted bodily functions, unsatisfying interpersonal relationships, and behaviors that interfere with routine functioning. Examples of psychoneurotic disorders that are described in the *DSM-IV-TR* include anxiety disorders, somatoform disorders, and dissociative disorders (discussed in Chapters 16 and 17).

(5) Extended periods of functioning at the panic level of anxiety may result in psychotic behavior. Psychoses are serious psychiatric disturbances characterized by the presence of delusions and/or hallucinations and the impairment of interpersonal functioning and relationship to the external world. Examples of psychotic responses to anxiety include the schizophrenic, schizoaffective, and delusional disorders (discussed in Chapter 14).

3. Grief
   a. Defined: The subjective state of emotional, physical, and social responses to the loss of a valued entity. The loss may be real or perceived.
   b. Kubler-Ross has identified five stages of the grief process through which individuals pass as a normal response to loss.
      (1) Denial—a stage of shock and disbelief.
      (2) Anger—that which is felt for experiencing the loss is displaced upon the environment or turned inward on the self.
      (3) Bargaining—promises made to God for delaying the loss.
      (4) Depression—the full impact of the loss is felt; disengagement from all association with the lost entity is initiated.
      (5) Acceptance—resignation that the loss has occurred; a feeling of peace regarding the loss is experienced.
   c. Anticipatory grief is the experiencing of the grief process prior to the actual loss.
   d. Resolution. Length of the grief process is entirely individual. It can last from a few weeks to years. It is influenced by a number of factors:
      (1) The experience of guilt for having had a "love-hate" relationship with the lost entity. Guilt often lengthens the grieving process.
      (2) **Anticipatory grieving** is thought to shorten the grief response when the loss actually occurs.

(3) The length of the grief response is often extended when an individual has experienced a number of recent losses and when he or she is unable to complete one grieving process before another one begins.

(4) Resolution of the grief response is thought to have occurred when an individual can look back on the relationship with the lost entity and accept both the pleasures and the disappointments (both the positive and the negative aspects) of the association.

e. Maladaptive grief responses

(1) Prolonged response is an intense preoccupation with memories of the lost entity for many years after the loss has occurred. Behavior is characterized by disorganization of functioning and intense emotional pain related to the lost entity.

(2) Delayed or inhibited response is a fixation in the denial stage of the grieving process. The loss is not experienced, but there may be evidence of psychophysiological or psychoneurotic disorders.

(3) Distorted response is a fixation in the anger stage of the grieving process. All the normal behaviors associated with grieving are exaggerated out of proportion to the situation. The individual turns the anger inward on the self and is consumed with overwhelming despair. Pathological depression is a distorted grief response (discussed in Chapter 15).

V. *The Diagnostic and Statistical Manual of Mental Disorders, 4th ed, Text Revision (DSM-IV-TR)* Multiaxial Evaluation System. From the psychiatric diagnostic manual, individuals are evaluated on five axes:

A. Axis I—clinical disorders and other conditions that may be a focus of clinical attention.

B. Axis II—personality disorders and mental retardation.

C. Axis III—general medical conditions.

D. Axis IV—psychosocial and environmental problems.

E. Axis V—global assessment of functioning rated on the Global Assessment of Functioning (GAF) Scale that measures an individual's psychological, social, and occupational functioning.

VI. Summary

VII. Review Questions

LEARNING ACTIVITIES

EGO DEFENSE MECHANISMS—DEFINITIONS

In the box below, circle the names of the ego defense mechanisms defined as follows. The names may be identified in either direction vertically, horizontally, or diagonally. Number one is completed as an example.

1. Feelings are transferred from one target to another that is considered less threatening or neutral.

2. A mechanism that is used to symbolically negate or cancel out a previous action or experience that one finds intolerable.
3. The separation of a thought or a memory from the feeling, tone, or emotions associated with it.
4. Refusal to acknowledge the existence of a real situation or the feelings associated with it.
5. The beliefs and values of another individual are internalized and symbolically become a part of the self, to the extent that the feeling of separateness or distinctness is lost.
6. An attempt to increase self-worth by acquiring certain attributes and characteristics of an individual one admires.
7. A retreat to an earlier level of development and the comfort measures associated with that level of functioning.
8. Covering up a real or perceived weakness by emphasizing a trait one considers more desirable.
9. The involuntary blocking of unpleasant feelings and experiences from one's awareness.
10. Feelings or impulses unacceptable to one's self are attributed to another person.
11. The voluntary blocking of unpleasant feelings and experiences from one's awareness.
12. Attempting to make excuses or formulate logical reasons to justify unacceptable feelings or behaviors.

R	A	T	I	N	T	R	O	J	E	C	T	I	O	N
A	L	O	M	E	N	E	N	A	T	R	N	A	M	O
T	B	N	A	T	I	O	N	R	O	E	B	U	S	I
I	U	O	N	O	T	T	U	N	I	G	A	T	N	T
O	S	I	U	R	A	M	I	S	S	R	N	O	R	A
N	N	S	N	O	I	T	A	S	N	E	P	M	O	C
A	O	S	D	S	E	S	N	O	M	S	R	S	T	I
L	I	E	O	S	T	O	I	E	R	S	O	N	I	F
I	R	R	I	A	R	T	C	D	E	I	J	O	N	I
Z	U	P	N	R	A	A	S	T	R	O	E	A	N	T
A	R	P	G	L	L	U	M	I	O	N	C	I	O	N
T	E	U	O	P	R	O	J	N	E	I	T	I	O	E
I	R	S	S	U	P	R	E	S	L	A	I	N	E	D
O	I	I	R	E	P	R	E	S	S	I	O	N	N	I
N	D	I	S	P	U	C	E	M	E	N	N	T	I	O

THE GRIEF RESPONSE

Kubler-Ross identified five stages of the grief response: denial, anger, bargaining, depression, and acceptance. Fill in the blank with the appropriate stage that describes the verbal or behavioral response.

1. "I never want to see you again!" _____
2. "Cancer. It can't be! You must have made a mistake!" _____
3. "At last I feel at peace with myself." _____
4. "I'll go to church every Sunday if I can

just live till my daughter grows up."

5. "I wish I had been a better mother." _____

6. "Why me? I don't deserve this!" _____

7. "I'm feeling much better today. I think I
should get a second opinion." _____

8. "I feel as though I'm betraying my family.
They depend on me so." _____

9. "If God will only let me live till Christmas.
I swear I won't ask for another thing." _____

10. "My family is ready, and so I can rest easy
now." _____

CLINICAL EXERCISE

Have students keep a record of ego defense mechanisms they observe being used. These may be identified in the clinical setting, with their classmates, or with families or friends. Have them share these observations in their student group.

TEST QUESTIONS

1. When an individual's stress response is sustained over a long period of time, the endocrine system involvement results in:
   - • a. Decreased resistance to disease
     b. Increased libido
     c. Decreased blood pressure
     d. Increased inflammatory response

2. John, a 39-year-old Italian American, lives in an ethnic community of Italian immigrants. He and most of his peers are of the lower socioeconomic class. Recently John was charged with an act of voyeurism. Which of the following individuals would be most likely to label John's behavior as mental illness?
     a. John's parents, who are ashamed of his behavior
     b. John's friends from his "Sons of Italy" social club
   - • c. John's employer who owns the company where he works
     d. John's wife, who feels she must protect their children.

3. Which of the following best describes the characteristics of panic level of anxiety?
     a. Decreased attention span, hypotension, mild muscle tension
     b. Frequent body changes, feeling of nervousness, enhanced learning
     c. Narrow perceptual field, decreased problem-solving ability, mild gastric upset
   - • d. Feeling of losing control, misperceptions of the environment

4. Anne tends to use the defense mechanism of displacement. Her husband, whom she loves very much, yells at her for not having dinner ready when he comes home from work. She is most likely to react by:
    a. Telling her husband he has no right to yell at her.
    - b. Yelling at their son for slouching in his chair.
    c. Burning dinner.
    d. Saying to her husband, "I'll try to do better tomorrow."

5. Nancy hates her mother, who paid little attention to Nancy when she was growing up. Nancy uses the defense mechanism of reaction formation. Which of the following statements represents this defense mechanism?
    a. "I don't like to talk about my relationship with my mother."
    b. "It's my mother's fault that I feel this way."
    - c. "I have a very wonderful mother whom I love very much."
    d. "My mom always loved my sister more than she loved me."

6. Jack and Jill were recently divorced. Jill was devastated by the divorce and became very depressed. She sought counseling at the community mental health center. Which of the following statements by Jill would indicate that she has resolved the grief over loss of her marriage?
    a. "I know things would be different if we could only try again."
    b. "He will be back. I know he will."
    c. "I'm sure I did lots of things to provoke his anger."
    - d. "Yes, it was a difficult relationship, and he abused the children and me."

7. Sarah's husband, Frank, died 23 years ago. She has not changed a thing in their house since he died. She still has all of Frank's clothing in his closet, and his house slippers are still beside the bed where they were when he died. Sarah talks about Frank unceasingly to anyone who will listen. Which of the following pathological grief responses is Sarah exhibiting?
    a. Inhibited
    - b. Prolonged
    c. Delayed
    d. Distorted

8. The main difference between neurotic and psychotic behavior is that people experiencing neuroses:
    a. Are unaware that they are experiencing distress.
    b. Are unaware that their behaviors are maladaptive.
    c. Are aware of possible psychological causes of their behavior.
    - d. Experience no loss of contact with reality.

9. In assigning diagnoses to clients, psychiatrists use a multiaxial evaluation system from the *DSM-IV-TR*. Axis II of the system represents which of the following?
    - a. Personality disorders and mental retardation

b. Psychosocial and environmental problems
c. General medical conditions
d. Clinical disorders and other conditions that may be a focus of clinical attention

10. The Global Assessment of Function (GAF) Scale measures:
    a. Personality characteristics.
    b. Introversion/extroversion tendencies.
 • c. Psychological, social, and occupational functioning.
    d. Level of anxiety.

CHAPTER 2. CONCEPTS OF PERSONALITY DEVELOPMENT

CHAPTER FOCUS

The focus of this chapter is to provide background information for understanding the development of the personality. Major components of five leading theories are presented.

LEARNIING OBJECTIVES

After reading this chapter, the student will be able to:
1. Define *personality*.
2. Identify the ways in which knowledge of personality development is relevant to nursing in the psychiatric/mental health setting.
3. Discuss the major components of the following developmental theories:
   a. Psychoanalytic theory—Freud
   b. Interpersonal theory—Sullivan
   c. Theory of psychosocial development—Erikson
   d. Theory of object relations development—Mahler
   e. A nursing model of interpersonal development—Peplau

KEY TERMS

ego
id
superego
libido
personality
surrogate
temperament
psychodynamic nursing
counselor
technical expert

CHAPTER OUTLINE/LECTURE NOTES
I. Introduction
   A. **Personality** is defined by the *DSM-IV-TR* as "enduring patterns of perceiving, relating to, and thinking about the environment and oneself."
   B. Life-cycle developmentalists believe that people continue to development and change throughout life, thereby suggesting the possibility for renewal and growth in adults.
   C. Stages are identified by age. Personality is influenced by **temperament** (inborn personality characteristics) and the environment, however.
   D. It is possible for behaviors from an unsuccessfully completed stage to be modified and corrected in a later stage.

E. Stages overlap, and individuals may be working on tasks from more than one stage at a time.

F. Individuals may become fixed in a certain stage and remain developmentally delayed.

G. The *DSM-IV-TR* states that personality *disorders* occur when personality traits become inflexible and maladaptive, and cause either significant functional impairment or subjective distress.

II. Psychoanalytic Theory—S. Freud

   A. Freud believed basic character was formed by age 5 years.

   B. He organized the structure of the personality into three major components.

      1. **Id**. Present at birth, the id serves to satisfy needs and achieve immediate gratification. It has been called the "pleasure principle."

      2. **Ego**. Development begins at age 4 to 6 months. It serves as the rational part of the personality and works to maintain harmony between the external world, the id, and the **superego**. It is also called the "reality principle."

      3. Superego. Development begins at about 3 to 6 years. It is composed of the ego-ideal (the self-esteem that is developed in response to positive feedback) and the conscience (the culturally-influenced sense of right and wrong). May be referred to as the "perfection principle."

   C. Topography of the mind. Freud classified all mental contents and operations into three categories: the conscious, the preconscious, and the unconscious.

      1. The *conscious* includes all memories that remain within an individual's awareness.

      2. The *preconscious* includes all memories that may have been forgotten or are not in present awareness but that with attention can be readily recalled into consciousness.

      3. The *unconscious* includes all memories that one is unable to bring to conscious awareness.

   D. Dynamics of the personality

      1. Freud termed the force required for mental functioning *psychic energy*. It is transferred through all three components of the personality as the individual matures. If an excess of psychic energy is stored in one part of the personality, the behavior reflects that part of the personality.

      2. Freud termed the process by which the id invests energy into an object in an attempt to achieve gratification *cathexis*. *Anticathexis* is the use of psychic energy by the ego and the superego to control id impulses.

   E. Development of the personality. Freud identified five stages of development and the major developmental tasks of each.

      1. Oral stage (Birth to 18 months)—relief from anxiety through oral gratification of needs.

      2. Anal stage (18 months to 3 years)—learning independence and control, with focus on the excretory function.

      3. Phallic stage (3 to 6 years)—identification with parent of same sex; development of sexual identity; focus on genital organs.

4. Latency stage (6 to 12 years)—sexuality repressed; focus on relationships with same-sex peers.
5. Genital stage (13 to 20 years)—**libido** is reawakened as genital organs mature; focus on relationships with members of the opposite sex.

   F. Relevance to nursing practice. Being able to recognize behaviors associated with the id, ego, and superego will assist in the assessment of developmental level in clients. Understanding the use of ego defense mechanisms is important in making determinations about maladaptive behaviors and in planning care for clients to assist in creating change.

III. Interpersonal Theory—H.S. Sullivan
   A. Sullivan believed that individual behavior and personality development are the direct result of interpersonal relationships. The major components of this theory include:
1. Anxiety—viewed as a feeling of emotional discomfort, the relief or prevention of which is the aim of all behavior.
2. Satisfaction of needs—fulfillment of all requirements associated with an individual's physiochemical environment.
3. Interpersonal security—the feeling associated with relief from anxiety.
4. Self-system—a collection of experiences, or security measures, adopted by the individual to protect against anxiety; consists of three components:
   a. The "good me"—the part of the personality that develops in response to positive feedback.
   b. The "bad me"—the part of the personality that develops in response to negative feedback.
   c. The "not me"—the part of the personality that develops in response to situations that produce intense anxiety in the child.

   B. Stages of development. Sullivan identified six developmental stages and the major tasks associated with each.
1. Infancy (Birth to 18 months)—relief from anxiety through oral gratification of needs.
2. Childhood (18 months to 6 years)—learning to experience a delay in personal gratification without undue anxiety.
3. Juvenile (6 to 9 years)—learning to form satisfactory peer relationships.
4. Preadolescence (9 to 12 years)—learning to form satisfactory relationships with persons of same sex; the initiation of feelings of affection for another person.
5. Early adolescence (12 to 14 years)—learning to form satisfactory relationships with persons of the opposite sex; developing a sense of identity.
6. Late adolescence (14 to 21 years)—establishing self-identity; experiencing satisfying relationships; working to develop a lasting, intimate opposite-sex relationship.

   C. Relevance to nursing practice. Relationship development is a major psychiatric nursing intervention. Knowledge about the behaviors associated with all levels of anxiety and methods for alleviating anxiety helps nurses to assist clients achieve interpersonal security and a sense of well-being.

IV. Theory of Psychosocial Development—E. Erikson
   A. Erikson's theory is based on the influence of social processes on the development of the personality.
   B. Stages of development. Erikson identified eight stages of development and the major tasks associated with each.
      1. Infancy (Birth to 18 months)—trust versus mistrust; to develop a trust in the mothering figure and be able to generalize it to others. Failure results in emotional dissatisfaction with self and others, suspiciousness, and difficulty with interpersonal relationships.
      2. Early childhood (18 months to 3 years)—autonomy versus shame and doubt; to gain some self-control and independence within the environment. Failure results in a lack of self-confidence, a lack of pride in the ability to perform, a sense of being controlled by others, and a rage against the self.
      3. Late childhood (3 to 6 years)—initiative versus guilt; to develop a sense of purpose and the ability to initiate and direct one's own activities. Failure results in feelings of inadequacy and guilt and the accepting of liability in situations for which one is not responsible.
      4. School age (6 to 12 years)—industry versus inferiority; to achieve a sense of self-confidence by learning, competing, performing successfully, and receiving recognition from significant others, peers, and acquaintances. Failure results in difficulty in interpersonal relationships caused by feelings of inadequacy.
      5. Adolescence (12 to 20 years)—identity versus role confusion; to integrate the tasks mastered in the previous stages into a secure sense of self. Failure results in a sense of self-consciousness, doubt, and confusion about one's role in life.
      6. Young adulthood (20 to 30 years)—intimacy versus isolation; to form an intense, lasting relationship or a commitment to another person, a cause, an institution, or a creative effort. Failure results in withdrawal, social isolation, aloneness, and the inability to form lasting, intimate relationships.
      7. Adulthood (30 to 65 years)—generativity versus stagnation; to achieve the life goals established for oneself, while also considering the welfare of future generations. Failure results in lack of concern for the welfare of others and total preoccupation with the self.
      8. Old age (65 years to death)—ego integrity versus despair; to review one's life and derive meaning from both positive and negative events while achieving a positive sense of self-worth. Failure results in a sense of self-contempt and disgust with how life has progressed.
   C. Relevance to nursing practice. Many individuals with mental health problems are still struggling to achieve tasks from a number of developmental stages. Nurses can plan care to assist these individuals to fulfill these tasks and move on to a higher developmental level.
V. Theory of Object Relations—M. Mahler
   A. Mahler's theory is based on the separation-individuation process of the infant from the maternal figure (primary caregiver).

B. Stages of development. Mahler identified six phases and subphases through which the individual progresses on the way to object constancy. Major developmental tasks are also described.

    1. Phase I. Normal autism (Birth to 1 month)—fulfillment of basic needs for survival and comfort. Fixation at this level can predispose to autistic disorder.

    2. Phase II. Symbiosis (1 to 5 months)—developing awareness of external source of need fulfillment. Lack of expected nurturing in this phase may lead to symbiotic psychosis.

    3. Phase III. Separation-individuation—the process of separating from mothering figure and the strengthening of the sense of self. Divided into four subphases:

        a. Subphase 1—differentiation. Beginning of a primary recognition of separateness from the mother.

        b. Subphase 2—practicing. Increased independence through locomotor functioning; increased sense of separateness of self.

        c. Subphase 3—rapprochement. Acute awareness of separateness of self; learning to seek "emotional refueling" from mothering figure to maintain feeling of security.

        d. Subphase 4—consolidation. Sense of separateness established; on the way to object constancy: able to internalize a sustained image of loved object or person when it is out of sight; resolution of separation anxiety.

C. Relevance to nursing practice. Understanding the concepts of Mahler's theory of object relations assists the nurse to assess the client's level of individuation from primary caregivers. The emotional problems of many individuals can be traced to lack of fulfillment of the tasks of separation/individuation.

VI. A Nursing Model of Interpersonal Development—H. Peplau

A. Peplau applies the interpersonal theory to nurse-client relationship development.

B. Peplau correlates the stages of personality development in childhood to stages through which clients advance during the progression of an illness.

C. Interpersonal experiences are seen as learning situations for nurses to facilitate forward movement in the development of personality.

D. Peplau identifies six nursing roles in which nurses function to assist individuals in need of health services:

    1. Resource person—one who provides specific information.

    2. **Counselor**—one who listens while the client relates difficulties he or she is experiencing in any aspect of life.

    3. Teacher—one who identifies learning needs and provides information to client or family to fulfill those needs.

    4. Leader—one who guides the interpersonal interactions and ensures the fulfillment of goals.

    5. **Technical expert**—one who possesses the skills necessary to perform the interventions directed at improvement in the client's condition.

    6. **Surrogate**—one who serves as a substitute figure for another.

E. Peplau identifies four stages of personality development.

1. Stage 1—learning to count on others; the infant stage of development; learning to communicate in various ways with the primary caregiver in order to have comfort needs fulfilled.
2. Stage 2—learning to delay gratification; the toddlerhood stage of development; learning the satisfaction of pleasing others by delaying self-gratification in small ways.
3. Stage 3—identifying oneself; the early childhood stage of development; learning appropriate roles and behaviors by acquiring the ability to perceive the expectations of others.
4. Stage 4—developing skills in participation; the late childhood stage of development; learning the skills of compromise, competition, and cooperation with others; establishment of a more realistic view of the world and a feeling of one's place in it.

F. Relevance to nursing practice. Peplau's model provides nurses with a framework to interact with clients, many of whom are fixed in, or because of illness have regressed to, an earlier level of development. Using nursing roles suggested by Peplau, nurses may facilitate client learning to that which has not been learned in earlier experiences.

VII. Summary
VIII. Review Questions

LEARNING ACTIVITIES

Id, Ego, and Superego

Identify whether each of the behaviors described below is being directed by the id, ego, or superego components of the personality.

_____ 1. Mary stole some makeup off the shelf at the department store.

_____ 2. Mary began to feel very guilty for taking the makeup after she got home with it.

_____ 3. Mary took the makeup back to the store and apologized to the clerk for taking it.

_____ 4. Two-year-old Sandy has a temper tantrum when her Mother takes a dangerous toy away from her.

_____ 5. Sandy sucks on her thumb for comfort.

_____ 6. Frankie wants to do well on the algebra test and stays home to study instead of going out with his friends.

_____ 7. Frankie does not do as well on the algebra test as he had hoped. He becomes despondent and refuses to come out of his room for days.

_____ 8. Jack joins his friends when they invite him to drink beer and smoke marijuana with them.

_____ 9. After having a few beers, Jack decides not to drive his car home.

_____ 10. Jack tells his parents he is sorry for drinking beer and smoking marijuana.

Behaviors Identified by Erikson's Stages of Development

Match the behaviors or statements described on the right with Erikson's stages of development listed on the left. Both achievement and non-achievement are reflected in the choices.

_____ 1. Trust   a. "I don't like people. I'd rather be alone."

_____ 2. Mistrust   b. "Get away from me with that medicine. I know you are trying to poison me!"

_____ 3. Autonomy   c. "I feel good about my life. I have a lot to be thankful for."

_____ 4. Shame and Doubt   d. Five-year-old girl believes she is the cause of her parents' divorce.

_____ 5. Initiative   e. "Sure, I'll loan you $10 till your next payday."

_____ 6. Guilt   f. "I don't know what I want to do with my life. College? Work? What kind of job would I get anyway?"

_____ 7. Industry   g. "Mommy! Mommy! I made all A's on my report card!"

_____ 8. Inferiority   h. "I'll have to ask my husband. He's the decision maker in our family."

_____ 9. Identity   i. "When I graduate from college, I want to work with handicapped children."

_____ 10. Role Confusion   j. "I plan to work as hard as necessary to help women achieve equality. I plan to see this happens before I die."

_____ 11. Intimacy   k. "I hate this place. No one cares what I do anyway. It's just a way to bring home a paycheck."

_____12. Isolation   l. "Look, Mom! I ironed this blouse all by myself!"

_____13. Generativity   m. "If only I could live my life over again. I'd do things so much differently. I feel like a nothing."

_____14. Stagnation   n. "I could never be a nurse. I'm not smart enough."

_____15. Ego Integrity   o. "Yes, I will be the chairperson for the cancer drive."

_____16. Despair   p. "I have been the Girl Scout leader for Troop 259 for 7 years now."

TEST QUESTIONS

Please answer the questions based on the following case study.

Mrs. K. is 78 years old. She has been admitted to the psychiatric unit of a large hospital because she is depressed and told her daughter she no longer had anything to live for. She threatened to swallow her whole bottle of antihypertensive medication.

Mrs. K. lives alone. She has been married and divorced five times. She told the nurse, "Every time I got married, I thought it was for the rest of my life; but every time, we just couldn't get along. I like to be independent. I want to do what I want to do, when I want to do it, and I don't want some man getting in my way! Men are all alike. They think they own their wives. Well, not me!"

On the unit, Mrs. K. is quarrelsome with the other clients. She changes the TV channel to what she wants to watch without consulting the group; in group therapy, when the focus is on another person, she interrupts to discuss her own situation; and most of the time, she prefers to stay in her room alone, rather than interact with the other clients. She states, "Nobody wants to have anything to do with me, anyway. If I had my life to live over again, I'd sure do a lot of things differently."

1. _Theoretically_, in which level of psychosocial development (according to Erikson) would you place Mrs. K?
    a. Trust versus mistrust
    b. Industry versus inferiority
    c. Generativity versus stagnation
    • d. Ego integrity versus despair

2. According to Erikson's theory, where would you place Mrs. K. based on her behavior?
    a. Trust versus mistrust
    • b. Industry versus inferiority
    c. Generativity versus stagnation
    d. Ego integrity versus despair

3. In what stage of development is Mrs. K. fixed according to Sullivan's interpersonal theory?
   - a. Infancy. She relieves anxiety through oral gratification.
   - • b. Childhood. She has not learned to delay gratification.
   - c. Early adolescence. She is struggling to form an identity.
   - d. Late adolescence. She is working to develop a lasting relationship.

4. Which of the following describes the psychoanalytical structure of Mrs. K.'s personality?
   - a. Weak id, strong ego, weak superego
   - b. Strong id, weak ego, weak superego
   - c. Weak id, weak ego, punitive superego
   - • d. Strong id, weak ego, punitive superego

5. In which of Peplau's stages of development would you assess Mrs. K?
   - a. Learning to count on others
   - • b. Learning to delay gratification
   - c. Identifying oneself
   - d. Developing skills in participation

General questions related to theories of personality development.

6. According to Mahler's theory, feelings of rage and fear of abandonment that may persist into adulthood can occur when a child becomes fixed in what stage of development?
   - • a. Rapprochement
   - b. Practicing
   - c. Differentiation
   - d. Autistic phase

7. According to Erikson's theory, which of the following is an example of nonachievement of the tasks associated with the stage of ego integrity versus despair?
   - a. "Daddy left us because I was a very bad girl."
   - b. "You have to look out for 'Number One.' Everyone's out to take all they can get from you."
   - c. "Why should I give a donation? No one ever gave me anything!"
   - • d. "My life was such a bummer! Seems like I failed at everything I tried to do!"

8. Freud believed that unsuccessful completion of which of the following stages of development results in traits such as stinginess, stubbornness, and untidiness?
   - a. Oral stage
   - • b. Anal stage
   - c. Phallic stage

d. Genital stage

9. "Emotional refueling" is a term used by Mahler in her theory of personality development. Which of the following best identifies this term?
    a. With advanced locomotor functioning, the child experiences feelings of exhilaration from increased independence.
    b. A type of psychic fusion of mother and child.
  • c. A fulfillment by the mothering figure of the child's emotional needs as required.
    d. The achievement of separation/individuation on the part of the child.

10. Peplau identified "surrogate" as one of the functional roles of the nurse. Which of the following statements is indicative of the surrogate role?
    a. "I will give you a tour of the unit after we complete the intake interview."
    b. "These are the possible side effects of the medication you will be taking."
    c. "Tell me about the relationship you had with your father."
  • d. "That type of behavior is not acceptable. I am committed to helping you succeed in this rehabilitation program."

CHAPTER 3. BIOLOGICAL IMPLICATIONS

CHAPTER FOCUS

The focus of this chapter is to explore the role of neurophysiological, neurochemical, and endocrine influences on psychiatric illness. Various diagnostic procedures used to detect alteration in biological function that may contribute to psychiatric illness are identified, and the implications to psychiatric/mental health nursing are discussed.

LEARNING OBJECTIVES

After reading this chapter the student will be able to:
1. Identify gross anatomical structures of the brain and describe their functions.
2. Discuss the physiology of neurotransmission within the central nervous system.
3. Describe the role of neurotransmitters in human behavior.
4. Discuss the association of endocrine functioning to the development of psychiatric disorders.
5. Discuss the correlation of alteration in brain functioning to various psychiatric disorders.
6. Identify various diagnostic procedures used to detect alteration in biological functioning that may be contributing to psychiatric disorders.
7. Discuss the implications of psychobiological concepts to the practice of psychiatric/mental health nursing.

KEY TERMS

limbic system
neurons
axon
dendrites
synapse
neurotransmitters
receptor sites
neuroendocrine system
cell body

CHAPTER OUTLINE/LECTURE NOTES

I. Introduction
   A. The 101st legislature of the United States designated the 1990s as the "decade of the brain" with the challenge of studying the biological basis of behavior.
   B. In keeping with the "neuroscientific revolution," greater emphasis has been placed on the study of the organic basis for psychiatric illness.
II. Nervous System

A. Central nervous system
   1. The brain
      a. The cerebrum
         (1) Consists of a right and left hemisphere connected by a deep groove of **neurons** (nerve cells) called the *corpus callosum*.
         (2) The cerebral *cortex* (or outer shell) is extensively folded and consists of billions of neurons.
         (3) Each hemisphere is divided into four lobes, each named for the overlying bones in the cranium: the frontal lobe, parietal lobe, temporal lobe, and occipital lobe.
            (a) Frontal lobes are responsible for voluntary body movement, including movements that permit speaking, thinking and judgment formation, and expression of feelings.
            (b) Parietal lobes are responsible for perception and interpretation of most sensory information (including touch, pain, taste, and body position).
            (c) Temporal lobes are responsible for hearing, short-term memory, and sense of smell; also responsible for expression of emotions through connection with the **limbic system**.
            (d) Occipital lobes are responsible for visual reception and interpretation.
      b. Diencephalon
         (1) The diencephalon connects the cerebrum with the lower brain structures and consists of the thalamus, hypothalamus, and limbic system.
         (2) The thalamus integrates all sensory input (except smell) on the way to the cortex; also has some involvement with emotions and mood.
         (3) The hypothalamus regulates anterior and posterior lobes of the pituitary gland and exerts control over actions of the autonomic nervous system. Also regulates appetite and temperature.
         (4) The limbic system consists of medially placed cortical and subcortical structures and the fiber tracts connecting them with one another and with the hypothalamus. It is sometimes call the "emotional brain" and is associated with feelings of fear and anxiety; anger and aggression; love, joy, and hope; and with sexuality and social behavior.
      c. Mesencephalon. The mesencephalon, or midbrain, is responsible for visual, auditory, and balance ("righting") reflexes.
      d. Pons. The pons is charged with regulation of respiration and skeletal muscle tone; ascending and descending tracts connect brainstem with cerebellum and cortex.
      e. Medulla. The medulla is a pathway for all ascending and descending fiber tracts. It contains vital centers that regulate heart rate, blood pressure, and respiration; reflex centers for swallowing, sneezing, coughing, and vomiting.

f. Cerebellum. The cerebellum regulates muscle tone and coordination and maintains posture and equilibrium.

2. Nerve tissue

    a. Neurons

        (1) The nerve cells of CNS tissue are called neurons and are composed of 3 parts: a **cell body**, an **axon**, and **dendrites**.

        (2) The cell body contains the nucleus and is essential for the life of the neuron.

        (3) The axon transmits impulses away from the cell body.

        (4) The dendrites are processes that transmit impulses toward the cell body.

        (5) Three classes of neurons exist within the CNS: afferent (sensory), efferent (motor), and interneurons.

            (a) Afferent neurons carry impulses from receptors in the internal and external periphery to the CNS, where they are interpreted into various sensations.

            (b) Efferent neurons carry impulses from the CNS to muscles (which respond by contracting) and glands (which respond by secreting).

            (c) Interneurons exist entirely within the CNS. They may carry only sensory or motor impulses, or they may serve as integrators in the pathways between afferent and efferent neurons.

    b. Synapses

        (1) The junction between two neurons is called a **synapse,** and the small space between the two neurons is called a synaptic cleft. Neurons conducting impulses toward the synapse are called presynaptic neurons, and those conducting impulses away are called postsynaptic neurons.

        (2) A chemical neurotransmitter is stored in the axon terminals of the presynaptic neuron. An electrical impulse causes its release into the synaptic cleft, where it combines with **receptor sites** on the postsynaptic neuron and determines whether or not another electrical impulse will be generated.

    c. Neurotransmitters

        (1) **Neurotransmitters** play an important role in human emotions and behavior and are the target for the mechanism of action in many psychotropic medications.

        (2) Neurotransmitters are stored in terminal vesicles of neuronal axons. When an electrical impulse reaches this point, the neurotransmitter is released from the vesicles into the synaptic cleft, where it binds with receptor sites on the postsynaptic neuron to determine whether or not another electrical impulse will be generated. After the neurotransmitter has accomplished this task, it is either inactivated and dissolved by enzymes or returned to the vesicles to be stored and used again.

(3) Major categories of neurotransmitters include cholinergics, monoamines, amino acids, and neuropeptides.

    (a) Cholinergics: Acetylcholine is found in the cerebral cortex, hippocampus, limbic structures, and basal ganglia. It is involved in sleep, arousal, pain perception, movement, and memory. It may be implicated in certain disorders of motor behavior and memory, as well as in depression.

    (b) Monoamines

        (i) Norepinephrine is found in the thalamus, hypothalamus, limbic system, hippocampus, cerebellum, and cerebral cortex. It influences mood, cognition, perception, locomotion, cardiovascular functioning, and sleep and arousal.

        (ii) Dopamine is found in the frontal cortex, limbic system, basal ganglia, thalamus, posterior pituitary, and spinal cord. It is involved in movement and coordination, emotions, voluntary judgment, and release of prolactin. It may be implicated in mood disorders and schizophrenia.

        (iii) Serotonin is found in the hypothalamus, thalamus, limbic system, cerebral cortex, cerebellum, and spinal cord. It influences sleep and arousal, libido, appetite, mood, aggression, pain perception, coordination, and judgment.

        (iv) Histamine is found in the hypothalamus. Its exact function is unclear but may have some influence on mood.

    (c) Amino acids

        (i) Gamma aminobutyric acid (GABA) is found in the hypothalamus, hippocampus, cortex, cerebellum, ganglia, spinal cord, and retina. It is involved in the slowdown of body activity.

        (ii) Glycine is found in the spinal cord and brainstem. It causes recurrent inhibition of motor neurons.

        (iii)Glutamate and aspartate are found in pyramidal cells of the cortex, cerebellum, and the primary sensory afferent systems; also the hippocampus, thalamus, hypothalamus, and spinal cord. They are involved in the relay of sensory information and in the regulation of various motor and spinal reflexes.

    (d) Neuropeptides

        (i) Endorphins and enkephalins are found in the hypothalamus, thalamus, limbic structures, midbrain, and brainstem. Enkephalins are also found in the GI tract. They are involved in the modulation of pain and the reduction of peristalsis (enkephalins).

(ii) Substance P is found in the hypothalamus, limbic structures, midbrain, brainstem, thalamus, basal ganglia, and spinal cord. Also found in the GI tract and salivary glands. It is involved in the regulation of pain.

(iii) Somatostatin is found in the cerebral cortex, hippocampus, thalamus, basal ganglia, brainstem, and spinal cord. It inhibits release of serotonin, dopamine, and acetylcholine.

3. Spinal cord

    a. Fiber Tracts. Around the external part of the spinal cord is an area of white matter, so called because the fibers that make up the area are sheathed in a white, lipid substance called myelin. The gray matter in the center is made up of the cell bodies of motor neurons and interneurons. Ascending spinal tracts carry sensory impulses to the brain and descending tracts carry motor impulses from the brain to the periphery.

    b. Spinal nerves. There are 31 pairs of spinal nerves that are identified by the level of the vertebrae from which they arise.

      (1) Cervical nerves supply the upper portion of the body, including the diaphragm.

      (2) Thoracic nerves supply the trunk of the body.

      (3) Lumbar and sacral nerves supply the hips, pelvic cavity, and legs.

B. Peripheral nervous system

    1. The afferent system. Afferent, or sensory, neurons convey information from receptors in the periphery to the CNS.

      a. Somatic sensory neurons originate from external areas of the body, such as skin, skeletal muscles, and joints.

      b. Visceral sensory neurons originate from receptors in internal organs.

    2. The efferent system. Efferent, or motor, neurons carry information from the CNS to peripheral areas of the body, namely skeletal muscles, smooth and cardiac muscles, and glands. The efferent system is made up of two major systems: the somatic nervous system and the autonomic nervous system (ANS).

      a. The somatic nervous system consists of fibers that go from the central nervous system (either brain or spinal cord) to skeletal muscles cells and are responsible for the contraction of skeletal muscle. These neurons are sometimes called somatic motor neurons.

      b. ANS neurons (sometimes called visceral motor neurons) innervate smooth muscles, cardiac muscles and glands. The ANS is further divided into *sympathetic* and *parasympathetic* components. When the activity of one of these components is enhanced, the activity of the other is suppressed.

        (1) The sympathetic nervous system is activated during stressful situations and prepares the body for "fight or flight." Acetylcholine and norepinephrine are the major neurotransmitters of this system.

        (2) The parasympathetic nervous system is dominant in the non-stressful or relaxed state. The neurotransmitter found in the parasympathetic nervous system is acetylcholine.

III. **Neuroendocrine System**: Pituitary Gland
  A. Endocrine functioning in the CNS is under the influence of the hypothalamus, which has direct control over the pituitary gland, sometimes called the "master gland."
  B. The pituitary gland has two major lobes, the posterior lobe (also called the neurohypophysis) and the anterior lobe (also called the adenohypophysis).
    1. The posterior lobe is under neural control of the hypothalamus. Two hormones, vasopressin (or ADH) and oxytocin, are produced in the hypothalamus and stored in the posterior pituitary. Their release is mediated by neural impulses from the hypothalamus.
       a. ADH conserves body water and maintains normal blood pressure. Its release is stimulated by pain, emotional stress, dehydration, increased plasma concentration, and decreases in blood volume.
       b. Oxytocin stimulates contraction of the uterus at the end of pregnancy and stimulates release of milk from the mammary glands. Its role in behavioral functioning is unclear.
    2. The anterior lobe produces a number of hormones whose release is under the control of releasing hormones that are produced by the hypothalamus. When these pituitary hormones are required by the body, the releasing hormones from the hypothalamus pass through the capillaries and veins of the hypophyseal portal system to capillaries in the anterior pituitary, where they stimulate secretion of these specialized hormones.
       a. Growth hormone is responsible for growth in children and for continued protein synthesis throughout life. During prolonged stress, it has a direct effect on protein, carbohydrate, and lipid metabolism, resulting in increased serum glucose and free fatty acids to be used for increased energy.
       b. Thyroid-stimulating hormone stimulates the thyroid gland to secrete thyroid hormones necessary for metabolism of food and regulation of temperature.
       c. ACTH stimulates the adrenal cortex to secrete cortisol, which plays a role in the response to stress.
       d. Prolactin stimulates the breasts to produce milk.
       e. Gonadotropic hormones stimulate the ovaries and testes to secrete estrogen, progesterone, and testosterone. Estrogen and progesterone also play a role in ovulation, and testosterone plays a role in sperm production.
       f. Melanocyte-stimulating hormone stimulates the pineal gland to secrete melatonin, a hormone that may be implicated in the etiology of seasonal affective disorder (SAD).
IV. Implications for Psychiatric Illness
  A. Schizophrenia
    1. Anomalies of the brain: Several anatomical anomalies have been found within the brains of individuals with schizophrenia. They include:
       a. Enlarged ventricular size.
       b. Dilation of cortical sulci and fissures.
       c. Decreased temporal lobe size.
       d. Functional asymmetry related to language comprehension and speech

production.

      e. Histological changes in limbic system, thalamus, basal ganglia, hippocampus, and frontal cortex.

  2. Neurotransmitter hypothesis: Various biochemicals have been implicated in the etiology of schizophrenia.

      a. An excess of dopamine.

      b. Abnormalities in norepinephrine, serotonin, acetylcholine, GABA, prostaglandins, and endorphins also may be contributing factors.

  3. Possible endocrine correlation: There may be some correlation between decreased levels of the hormone prolactin and schizophrenia.

B. Mood disorders

  1. Neuroanatomical considerations: Symptoms of mood disorders, as well as biological research findings, support the hypothesis that mood disorders involve pathology of the limbic system, the basal ganglia, and the hypothalamus.

  2. Neurotransmitter hypothesis

      a. Symptoms of depression are associated with a deficiency of norepinephrine and dopamine.

      b. Symptoms of mania are associated with an excess of norepinephrine and dopamine.

      c. Serotonin appears to remain low in both states.

  3. Possible endocrine correlation: Several hormonal anomalies have been correlated with mood disorders. They include the following:

      a. In depression, the failure of normal hormonal inhibition results in a hypersecretion of cortisol.

      b. Hypothyroidism has been associated with symptoms of depression and hyperthyroidism with acute mania.

      c. Increased secretion of melatonin from the pineal gland has been correlated with SAD.

C. Anxiety disorders

  1. Neuroanatomical considerations: Pathology in various areas of the brain has been correlated with symptoms of anxiety disorders. These include the following:

      a. Stimulation of the limbic system produces anxiety and fear responses.

      b. The cingulate gyrus of the limbic system and the temporal cortex have been implicated in the pathophysiology of obsessive-compulsive disorder.

  2. Neurotransmitter hypothesis

      a. Elevated levels of norepinephrine are implicated in the etiology of panic disorder.

      b. Serotonin may play a role in the behaviors associated with obsessive-compulsive disorder.

      c. Inhibition of the neurotransmitter GABA is associated with elevated levels of anxiety.

  3. Possible endocrine correlation

      a. Increased levels of thyroid-stimulating hormone and prolactin have been observed in individuals with anxiety disorders.

      b. Some individuals with obsessive-compulsive disorder exhibit increased cortisol levels.

D. Anorexia nervosa

    1. Neuroanatomical considerations: Some individuals with anorexia nervosa have exhibited a reversible phenomenon of enlarged sulci and ventricles during the starvation period.

    2. Neurotransmitter hypothesis: Decreased levels of norepinephrine, serotonin, and dopamine have been correlated with eating disorders.

    3. Possible endocrine correlation: A possible primary hypothalamic dysfunction has been associated with anorexia nervosa.

E. Alzheimer's disease

    1. Neuroanatomical considerations

      a. Observation of a brain from an individual with Alzheimer's disease reveals diffuse atrophy with flattened cortical sulci and enlarged cerebral ventricles.

      b. Microscopic findings include senile plaques, neurofibrillary tangles, and neuronal loss.

    2. Neurotransmitter hypothesis

      a. There are decreased levels of acetylcholine in the cells of the cortex and hippocampus.

      b. There are decreased levels of norepinephrine and somatostatin.

    3. Possible endocrine correlation: The hormone corticotropin has been reported to be decreased in Alzheimer's disease.

V. Diagnostic Procedures Used to Detect Altered Brain Functioning

A. Electroencephalography (EEG)

    1. Electrodes are placed on the scalp to measure amplitude and frequency of brain waves.

    2. EEG is used to identify anomalies in brain rhythm and in the diagnosis of epilepsy, neoplasm, stroke, metabolic, or degenerative disease.

B. Computerized EEG mapping

    1. EEG tracings are summarized to identify functioning in various regions of the brain.

    2. They are used largely in research to represent statistical relationships between individuals and groups or between two populations of subjects.

C. Computed tomographic (CT) scan

    1. X-rays are taken of various transverse planes of the brain.

    2. A CT scan is used to detect possible lesions, abscesses, areas of infarction, or aneurysm. It is also used to identify anatomic differences in clients with schizophrenia, organic mental disorders, and bipolar disorder.

D. Magnetic resonance imaging (MRI)

    1. Within a strong magnetic field, the nuclei of hydrogen atoms absorb and re-emit electromagnetic energy that is computerized and transformed into image information.

2. MRI is used to detect brain edema, ischemia, infection, neoplasm, trauma, and other changes such as demyelination. Morphological differences have been noted in brains of clients with schizophrenia as compared with control subjects.

E. Positron emission tomography (PET)
1. A radioactive substance injected into the individual is then read by detectors that relay data to a computer, which interprets the signals and produces the image.
2. PET measures specific brain functioning, such as glucose metabolism, oxygen utilization, blood flow, and, of particular interest in psychiatry, neurotransmitter and receptor interaction.

F. Single photon emission computer tomography (SPECT)
1. This technique is similar to PET, but a longer-acting radioactive substance is used to allow time for a gamma camera to rotate about the head and gather the data.
2. SPECT is used to measure brain functioning and to image activity or cerebrospinal fluid (CSF) circulation.

VI. Implications for Nursing
A. Psychiatric nurses must integrate knowledge of the biological sciences into their practices if they are to ensure safe and effective care for people with mental illness.
B. To ensure a smooth transition from a psychosocial focus to one of biopsychosocial emphasis, nurses must have a clear understanding of the following:
1. Neuroanatomy and neurophysiology.
2. Neuronal processes.
3. Neuroendocrinology.
4. Circadian rhythms.
5. Genetic influences.
6. Psychoimmunology.
7. Psychopharmacology.
8. Diagnostic technology.

VII. Summary
VIII. Review Questions

TEST QUESTIONS

1. Which of the following cerebral structures is sometimes referred to as the "emotional brain?"
   a. The cerebellum
 • b. The limbic system
   c. The cortex

d. The left temporal lobe

Central nervous system nerve cells are called neurons and consist of three types. In questions 2, 3, and 4, match the cell type named on the left with its major function on the right.

2. __c__ Afferent neurons   a. Motor neurons that carry impulses from the CNS
                                          to muscles and glands of the periphery.

3. __a__ Efferent neurons   b. Serve as integrators between pathways and
                                          account in large part for thinking, feelings,
                                          learning, language, and memory.

4. __b__ Interneurons   c. Sensory neurons that carry impulses from the
                                          periphery to the CNS.

Neurotransmitters and hormones may play a significant role in psychiatric illness. In questions 5, 6, 7, and 8, match the neurotransmitters named on the left with the implication for psychiatric illness on the right.

5. __b__ Increased dopamine   a. Alzheimer's disease

6. __d__ Decreased norepinephrine b. Schizophrenia

7. __c__ Decreased GABA   c. Anxiety disorders

8. __a__ Decreased acetylcholine d. Depression

In questions 9, 10, and 11, match the hormones named on the left with the implication for psychiatric illness on the right.

9. __c__ Elevated CSF cortisol   a. Acute mania

10. __a__ Elevated thyroid hormone b. Schizophrenia

11. __b__ Decreased prolactin   c. Anorexia Nervosa

LEARNING ACTIVITIES

Label the parts indicated.

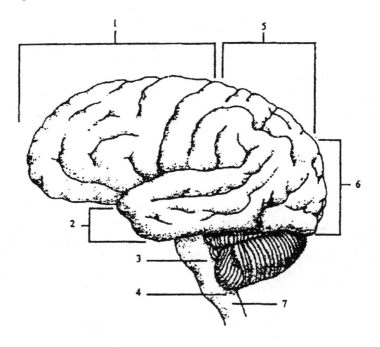

_____ Frontal lobe
_____ Parietal lobe
_____ Temporal lobe
_____ Occipital lobe

_____ Medulla
_____ Cerebellum
_____ Pons

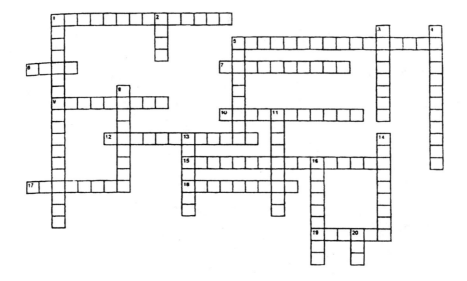

ACROSS

1. Neurotransmitter released in response to stress
5. Study of the implications of the immune system in psychiatry
6. Part of the neuron that carries impulses away from the cell body
7. Structure of the brain associated with muscular coordination and posture
9. Part of the neuron that carries impulses toward the cell body
10. Cells of the immune system
12. Sometimes called the "emotional brain" (two words)
15. Chemical stored in the axon terminals neurons
17. Part of the neuron that contains the nucleus (two words)
18. Hormone that stimulates breast milk production and may play a role in depression
19. A nerve cell

DOWN

1. The study of hormones functioning within the neurological system
2. Structure of the brain associated with regulation of respiration
3. Increased levels of this neurotransmitter are implicated in schizophrenia
4. Structure of the brain that controls pituitary function
5. The physical characteristics of a particular genotype
8. Sometimes called the "master gland"
11. Neurotransmitter that mediates allergic and inflammatory reactions
13. The junction between two neurons
14. Neurotransmitter thought to induce sleep and is decreased in depression
16. Hormone secreted by the pineal gland; implicated in the etiology of depression
20. Rapid eye movement; dream cycle sleep

CHAPTER 4. ETHICAL AND LEGAL ISSUES

CHAPTER FOCUS

The focus of this chapter is on ethical and legal issues that affect psychiatric/mental health nursing. Ethical theories, dilemmas, and principles are explored as a foundation for decision making. Various types of law are defined, and situations for which nurses may be held liable are discussed.

LEARNING OBJECTIVES

After reading this chapter, the student will be able to:
1. Differentiate among ethics, morals, values, and rights.
2. Discuss ethical theories including utilitarianism, Kantianism, Christian ethics, natural law theories, and ethical egoism.
3. Define *ethical dilemma*.
4. Discuss the ethical principles of autonomy, beneficence, nonmaleficence, and justice.
5. Use an ethical decision-making model to make an ethical decision.
6. Describe ethical issues relevant to psychiatric/mental health nursing.
7. Define *statutory law* and *common law*.
8. Differentiate between civil and criminal law.
9. Discuss legal issues relevant to psychiatric/mental health nursing.
10. Differentiate between *malpractice* and *negligence*.
11. Identify behaviors relevant to the psychiatric/mental health setting for which specific malpractice action could be taken.

KEY TERMS

assault	Kantianism
autonomy	libel
battery	malpractice
beneficence	moral behavior
bioethics	natural law
Christian ethics	negligence
civil law	nonmaleficence
common law	privileged communication
criminal law	right
defamation of character	slander
ethical dilemma	statutory law
ethical egoism	torts
ethics	utilitarianism
false imprisonment	values
informed consent	values clarification
justice	

CHAPTER OUTLINE/LECTURE NOTES

I. Introduction
   A. Nurses are constantly faced with the challenge of making difficult decisions regarding good and evil or life and death.
   B. Legislation determines what is "**right**" or "good" within a society.
II. Definitions
   A. **Ethics**—a branch of philosophy dealing with **values** related to human conduct, to the rightness and wrongness of certain actions, and to the goodness and badness of the motives and ends of such actions.
   B. **Bioethics**—applies to ethics when they refer to concepts within the scope of medicine, nursing, and allied health.
   C. **Moral behavior**—conduct that results from serious critical thinking about how individuals ought to treat others.
   D. Values—personal beliefs about the truth, beauty, or worth of a thought, object, or behavior.
   E. **Values clarification**—a process of self-discovery by which people identify their personal values and their value rankings.
   F. Right—that to which an individual is entitled (by ethical or moral standards) to have, or to do, or to receive from within the limits of the law.
   G. Absolute right—when there is no restriction whatsoever upon the individual's entitlement.
   H. Legal right—a right upon which the society has agreed and formalized into law.
III. Ethical Considerations
   A. Theoretical perspectives
      1. **Utilitarianism**—an ethical theory that promotes action based on the end results that produce the most good (happiness) for the most people.
      2. **Kantianism**—suggests that decisions and actions are bound by a sense of duty; also called *deontology*.
      3. **Christian ethics**—do unto others as you would have them do unto you; and alternatively, do not do unto others what you would not have them do unto you.
      4. **Natural law** theories--do good and avoid evil. Evil acts are never condoned, even if it is intended to advance the noblest of ends.
      5. **Ethical egoism**—decisions are based on what is best for the individual making the decision.
   B. **Ethical dilemmas**
      1. Ethical dilemmas occur when moral appeals can be made for taking each of two opposing courses of action.
      2. Taking no action is considered an action taken.
   C. Ethical principles
      1. **Autonomy**—principle emphasizes the status of persons as autonomous moral agents whose right to determine their destinies should always be respected.
      2. **Beneficence**—refers to one's duty to benefit or promote the good of others.

3. **Nonmaleficence**—abstaining from negative acts toward another, including acting carefully to avoid harm.
4. **Justice**—principle based on the notion of a hypothetical social contract between free, equal, and rational persons. The concept of justice reflects a duty to treat all individuals equally and fairly.
5. Veracity—refers to one's duty to always be truthful.

D. A model for making ethical decisions
1. Assessment.
2. Problem identification.
3. Plan.
   a. Explore the benefits and consequences of each alternative.
   b. Consider principles of ethical theories.
   c. Select an alternative.
4. Implementation: act on the decision made and communicate the decision to others.
5. Evaluation: evaluate outcomes.

E. Ethical issues in psychiatric/mental health nursing
1. The right to refuse medication
2. The right to the least restrictive treatment alternative

IV. Legal Considerations
A. Nurse Practice Act defines the legal parameters of professional and practical nursing.
B. Types of law.
1. **Statutory laws**—those that have been enacted by legislative bodies, such as a county or city council, state legislature, or the Congress of the United States
2. **Common law**—derived from decisions made in previous cases
C. Classifications within statutory and common law
1. **Civil law**—protects the private and property rights of individuals and businesses
   a. **Torts**—a violation of a civil law in which an individual has been wronged. Torts may be intentional or unintentional.
   b. **Contracts**—compensation or performance of the obligation set forth in the contract is sought.
2. **Criminal law**—provides protection from conduct deemed injurious to the public welfare
D. Legal issues in psychiatric/mental health nursing
1. Confidentiality and right to privacy
   a. Doctrine of **privileged communication**
2. **Informed consent**
3. Restraints and seclusion
   a. **False imprisonment**
4. Commitment issues
   a. Voluntary commitment
   b. Involuntary commitment
   c. Emergency commitments

          d. The mentally ill person in need of treatment
          e. Involuntary outpatient commitment
          f. The gravely disabled client
    E. Nursing liability
          1. **Malpractice** and **negligence**
          2. Types of lawsuits that occur in psychiatric nursing
              a. Breach of confidentiality
              b. **Defamation of character**
                  (1) **Libel**
                  (2) **Slander**
              c. Invasion of privacy
              d. **Assault** and **battery**
              e. False imprisonment
    F. Avoiding liability
          1. Practice within the scope of the Nurse Practice Act.
          2. Observe the hospital's and department's policy manuals.
          3. Measure up to established practice standards.
          4. Always put the client's rights and welfare first.
          5. Develop and maintain a good interpersonal relationship with each client and
             his or her family.
  V. Summary
 VI. Review Questions

LEARNING ACTIVITY

ETHICAL AND LEGAL ISSUES IN PSYCHIATRIC/MENTAL HEALTH NURSING

Identify the following key terms associated with ethical and legal issues in
psychiatric/mental health nursing with the descriptions or definitions listed below.

a. assault	j. Kantianism
b. battery	k. malpractice
c. beneficence	l. natural law
d. Christian ethics	m. nonmaleficence
e. torts	n. slander
f. common law	o. statutory law
g. libel	p. utilitarianism
h. ethical egoism	q. civil law
i. false imprisonment	r. criminal law

_____ 1. Ethical theory by which decisions are based on a sense of duty
_____ 2. Writing false and malicious information about a person
_____ 3. The touching of another person without consent
_____ 4. Provides protection from conduct deemed injurious to the public welfare
_____ 5. Abstaining from negative acts toward another, including acting carefully to
          avoid harm

_____ 6. An act resulting in a person's genuine fear and apprehension that he or she will be touched without consent

_____ 7. The theory on which decisions are based in which evil acts are never condoned, even if they are intended to advance the noblest of ends

_____ 8. A violation of a civil law in which an individual has been wronged

_____ 9. The ethical theory on which decisions are based that ensure the greatest happiness to the greatest number of people

_____ 10. The deliberate and unauthorized confinement of a person within fixed limits by the use of threat or force

_____ 11. The failure of a professional to perform or to refrain from performing in a manner in which a reputable member within the profession would be expected to do so

_____ 12. An ethical principle that refers to one's duty to benefit or promote the good of others

_____ 13. Law that has been enacted by legislative bodies

_____ 14. Verbalizing false and malicious information about a person

_____ 15. An ethical theory that espouses making decisions based on what is most advantageous for the person making the decision

_____ 16. Law that is derived from decisions made in previous cases

_____ 17. Law that protects the private and property rights of individuals and businesses

_____ 18. The ethical theory that espouses "Do unto others as you would have others do unto you"

TEST QUESTIONS

1. Raymond is a 54-year old man with chronic schizophrenia who is seen monthly by a community mental health nurse for administration of fluphenazine decanoate (Prolixin decanoate). Raymond refuses his medication at one regularly scheduled monthly visit. Which of the following interventions by the nurse is considered to be ethically appropriate?
   - a. Tell Raymond it is his right not to take the medication.
   - b. Tell Raymond that if he does not take his medication he will have to be hospitalized.
   - c. Arrange with a relative to add medication to Raymond's morning orange juice.
   - d. Call for help from Security to hold Raymond down while the shot is administered.

2. Raymond is eventually hospitalized because he has become highly agitated, physically aggressive and unable to communicate cooperatively. With the help of hospital Security and the police who brought him in, the ER nurse and resident apply leather restraints to Raymond's arms and legs against his very loud protests.

Raymond yells that he is going to sue. Under which of the following conditions is the staff protected?
- a. Raymond is a voluntary commitment and poses no danger to self or others.
- b. Raymond is a voluntary commitment, but poses a danger to self or others.
- c. Raymond is an involuntary commitment, but poses no danger to self or others.
- • d. Raymond is an involuntary commitment and poses a danger to self or others.

3. Raymond threatens to sue the physician and the nurse who restrained him for assault and battery. Which of the following conditions identifies the criteria for this offense (outside of an emergency situation)?
- a. The staff members become angry with Raymond and call him offensive names.
- • b. Raymond is touched (or fears being touched) without his consent.
- c. The nurse hides Raymond's clothes so he cannot leave.
- d. The nurse puts Raymond in restraints against his wishes.

4. The nurse states, "Well, I know Raymond is against us putting him in restraints, but if I ever get in this condition, I hope people would do the same for me." This is an example of which ethical philosophy?
- a. Kantianism
- b. Utilitarianism
- • c. Christian ethics
- d. Natural law ethics

5. In an effort to adhere to the principle of least-restrictive alternative, instead of putting Raymond in leather restraints, the nurse might have (with physician's order):
- • a. Given Raymond an injection of a major tranquilizer.
- b. Put Raymond in a locked room by himself.
- c. Told Raymond if he didn't calm down, he would be given an ECT treatment.
- d. Put Raymond in soft, Posey restraints, rather than leather restraints.

6. Nancy is a nurse on the oncology unit. Joe, her client has just returned from surgery. He has been diagnosed with terminal cancer. Joe's family does not think he should be told about his health status. Nancy decides to tell Joe anyway, because she believes it is her duty to do so. This is an example of which ethical philosophy?
- • a. Kantianism
- b. Utilitarianism
- c. Christian ethics
- d. Natural law ethics

Match the following nursing actions with the possible legal action with which the nurse may be charged:

___7. Jack is a voluntary admission. The nurse tells Jack that if he refuses to go to Group Therapy, she will put him in the Seclusion Room. Jack responds, "You do, and I'll sue."

a. Breach of confidentiality

___8. The nurse says to Jack, "You'd better do as I say, Jack, or you'll end up in restraints. I'll see to that!"

b. Assault

___9. Jack's employer calls the unit after hearing a rumor at work that Jack has been hospitalized on the psychiatric unit. The nurse says, "Yes, he's here, for all the good it is doing. He's an alcoholic, and he doesn't really want our help!"

c. Slander

___10. The nurse continues her tirade to the employer (above question) with, "I wouldn't be at all surprised if he isn't heavy into drugs; probably taking them and selling them."

d. False imprisonment

CHAPTER 5. RELATIONSHIP DEVELOPMENT AND THERAPEUTIC COMMUNICATION

CHAPTER FOCUS

The focus of this chapter is to describe the dynamics of a therapeutic nurse-client relationship. The student is introduced to the concept of communication. Verbal and nonverbal components of expression are described, and a discussion of therapeutic and nontherapeutic techniques is included.

LEARNING OBJECTIVES

After reading this chapter, the student will be able to:
1. Describe the relevance and dynamics of a therapeutic nurse-client relationship.
2. Identify goals of the nurse-client relationship.
3. Identify and discuss essential conditions for a therapeutic relationship to occur.
4. Describe the phases of relationship development and the tasks associated with each phase.
5. Identify types of preexisting conditions that influence the outcome of the communication process.
6. Define *territoriality, density,* and *distance* as components of the environment.
7. Identify components of nonverbal expression.
8. Describe therapeutic and nontherapeutic verbal communication techniques.
9. Describe active listening.
10. Discuss therapeutic feedback.

KEY TERMS

rapport	concrete thinking
confidentiality	unconditional positive regard
genuineness	empathy
sympathy	territoriality
density	intimate distance
paralanguage	personal distance
public distance	social distance

CHAPTER OUTLINE/LECTURE NOTES

I.   Introduction
    A. The nurse-client relationship is the foundation upon which psychiatric nursing is established.
    B. The *therapeutic interpersonal relationship* is the process by which nurses provide care for clients in need of psychosocial intervention.
II. The Therapeutic Nurse-Client Relationship

A. A therapeutic nurse-client relationship can only occur when each views the other as a unique human being. When this occurs, both participants have needs met by the relationship.

B. Therapeutic relationships are goal oriented and directed at learning and growth promotion.

C. Goals are often achieved through use of the problem-solving model.
   1. Identify the client's problem.
   2. Promote discussion of desired changes.
   3. Identify realistic changes.
   4. Discuss aspects that cannot be realistically changed and ways to cope more adaptively.
   5. Discuss alternative strategies for creating changes the client desires to make.
   6. Weigh the benefits and consequences of each alternative.
   7. Assist the client to select an alternative.
   8. Encourage the client to implement the change.
   9. Provide positive feedback for the client's attempts to create change.
   10. Assist the client to evaluate outcomes of the change and make modifications as required.

D. Therapeutic use of self
   1. Defined: The ability to use one's personality consciously and in full awareness in an attempt to establish relatedness and to structure nursing interventions.
   2. Nurse must possess self-awareness, self-understanding, and a philosophical belief about life, death, and the overall human condition.

III. Conditions Essential to Development of a Therapeutic Relationship
A. **Rapport**—implies special feelings on the part of both the client and the nurse based on acceptance, warmth, friendliness, common interest, a sense of trust, and a non-judgmental attitude.

B. **Trust**—implies a feeling of confidence in another person's presence, reliability, integrity, veracity, and sincere desire to provide assistance when requested.

C. **Respect**—implies the dignity and worth of an individual regardless of his or her unacceptable behavior. Carl Rogers called this **unconditional positive regard**.

D. **Genuineness**—refers to the nurse's ability to be open, honest, and "real" in interactions with the client. Genuineness implies congruence between what is felt and what is being expressed.

E. **Empathy**—a process wherein an individual is able to see beyond outward behavior and sense accurately another's inner experience at a given point in time. With empathy, the nurse's feelings remain on an objective level. It differs from **sympathy** in that with sympathy the nurse actually shares what the client is feeling and experiences a need to alleviate distress.

IV. Phases of a Therapeutic Nurse-Client Relationship
A. The preinteraction phase
   1. Obtain information about the client from chart, significant others, or other health team members.
   2. Examine one's own feelings, fears, and anxieties about working with a particular client.

B. The orientation (introductory) phase
   1. Create environment of trust and rapport.
   2. Establish contract for intervention.
   3. Gather assessment data.
   4. Identify client's strengths and weaknesses.
   5. Formulate nursing diagnoses.
   6. Set mutually agreeable goals.
   7. Develop a realistic plan of action for meeting the goals.
   8. Explore feelings of both client and nurse.
C. The working phase
   1. Maintain trust and rapport.
   2. Promote client's insight and perception of reality.
   3. Use problem-solving model to work toward achievement of established goals.
   4. Overcome resistance behaviors.
   5. Continuously evaluate progress toward goal attainment.
D. The termination phase
   1. Therapeutic conclusion of the relationship occurs when:
      a. Progress has been made toward attainment of the goals.
      b. A plan of action for more adaptive coping with future stressful situations has been established.
      c. Feelings about termination of the relationship are recognized and explored.
V. Interpersonal Communication
A. The impact of preexisting conditions—both sender and receiver bring certain preexisting conditions to the exchange that influence both the intended message and the way in which it is interpreted.
   1. Values, attitudes, and beliefs. Examples:
      a. Attitudes of prejudice are expressed through negative stereotyping.
      b. A person who values youth may dress and behave in a manner that is characteristic of one who is much younger.
   2. Culture or religion. Cultural mores, norms, ideas, and customs provide the basis for our way of thinking. Examples:
      a. Men who hug each other on the street give a different message in the Italian culture than they would in the American culture.
      b. Some messages about religion are conveyed by wearing crosses around one's neck or hanging crucifixes on the wall.
   3. Social status. High status persons often convey their high-power position with gestures. Examples: less eye contact, more relaxed posture, louder voice pitch, more frequent use of hands on hips, power dressing, greater height, and more distance when communicating with individuals considered to be of lower social status.
   4. Gender. Masculine and feminine gestures influence messages conveyed in communication with others. Examples: differences in posture and gender roles within various cultures.
   5. Age or developmental level. Examples:

    a. Developmental level communication is especially evident during adolescence, with words such as cool, groovy, awesome, and others.

    b. Sign language is a unique system of gestures used by individuals who are deaf or hearing impaired.

6. Environment in which the transaction takes place. **Territoriality**, **density**, and distance are aspects of environment that communicate messages.

    a. Territoriality—the innate tendency to own space. All individuals lay claim to certain areas as their own and feel safer in their own area.

    b. Density—the number of people within a given environmental space. Prolonged exposure to high-density situations elicits certain behaviors, such as aggression, stress, criminal activity, and hostility.

    c. Distance—the means by which various cultures use space to communicate.

        (1) **Intimate distance**—the closest distance that individuals will allow between themselves and others. In the United States, it is 0 to 18 inches.

        (2) **Personal distance**—interactions that are personal in nature, such as close conversations with friends. In the United States, it is 18 to 40 inches.

        (3) **Social distance**—conversations with strangers or acquaintances (for example, at a cocktail party). In the United States, it is 4 to 12 ft.

        (4) **Public distance**—speaking in public or yelling to someone some distance away. In the United States, the distance exceeds 12 ft.

B. Nonverbal Communication

1. Physical appearance and dress. The ways in which individuals dress or wear their hair convey a message to all who observe the appearance. Example: Unkempt appearance may give an impression to some people that the individual is sloppy and irresponsible.

2. Body movement and posture. The way in which an individual positions his or her body communicates messages regarding self-esteem, gender identity, status, and interpersonal warmth and coldness. Examples:

    a. Slumped posture or head and eyes pointed downward conveys a message of low self-esteem.

    b. Sitting with legs crossed at the thighs sometimes depicts feminine identity.

    c. Standing tall with head high and hands on hips indicates a superior status over the person being addressed.

    d. Warmth is conveyed by a smile, direct eye contact, and keeping the hands still.

3. Touch can elicit both negative and positive reactions, depending on cultural interpretation. Types of touch include the following:

    a. Functional-professional: impersonal, businesslike touch. Example: tailor-fitting a suit.

    b. Social-polite: impersonal, but affirming. Example: a handshake.

    c. Friendship-warmth: indicates a strong liking for another person. Example: laying one's hand upon the shoulder of another.

       d. Love-intimacy: conveys an emotional attachment or attraction for another person. Example: to engage in a strong, mutual embrace.

       e. Sexual arousal: an expression of physical attraction. Example: touching another in the genital region.

   4. Facial expressions.

       a. Next to human speech, facial expression is the primary source of communication.

       b. The face can give multiple messages, such as happiness, sadness, anger, surprise, doubt, fear, disgust.

   5. Eye behavior.

       a. Eyes have been called the "windows of the soul."

       b. Social and cultural rules dictate where we can look, when we can look, for how long we can look, and at whom we can look.

       c. Eye contact conveys a personal interest in the other person.

       d. Staring or gazing can make another feel very uncomfortable.

   6. Vocal cues or **paralanguage**.

       a. Paralanguage is the gestural component of the spoken word. It consists of pitch, tone, and loudness of spoken messages, the rate of speaking, expressively placed pauses, and emphasis assigned to certain words.

       b. *How* a message is verbalized can be as important as *what* is verbalized.

C. Therapeutic communication techniques

   1. Silence—allows the client to take control of the discussion, if he or she so desires.

   2. Accepting—conveys positive regard.

   3. Giving recognition—acknowledging; indicating awareness.

   4. Offering self—making oneself available.

   5. Giving broad openings—allows client to select the topic.

   6. Offering general leads—encourages client to continue.

   7. Placing the event in time or sequence—clarifying the relationship of events in time.

   8. Making observations—verbalizing what is observed or perceived.

   9. Encouraging description of perceptions—asking the client to verbalize what is being perceived.

  10. Encouraging comparison—asking client to compare similarities and differences in ideas, experiences, or interpersonal relationships.

  11. Restating—lets the client know whether an expressed statement has been understood or not.

  12. Reflecting—questions or feelings are referred back to the client so that they may be recognized and accepted.

  13. Focusing—taking notice of a single idea or even a single word.

  14. Exploring—delving further into a subject, idea, experience, or relationship.

  15. Seeking clarification and validation—striving to explain that which is vague and searching for mutual understanding.

  16. Presenting reality—clarifying misperceptions that the client may be expressing.

17. Voicing doubt—expressing uncertainty as to the reality of the client's perceptions.
18. Verbalizing the implied—putting into words what the client has only implied.
19. Attempting to translate words into feelings—putting into words the feelings that client has expressed only indirectly.
20. Formulating a plan of action—strives to prevent anger or anxiety from escalating to an unmanageable level the next time the stressor occurs.

D. Nontherapeutic communication techniques
1. Giving reassurance—may discourage client from further expression of feelings if he or she believes they will only be belittled.
2. Rejecting—refusing to consider the client's ideas or behavior.
3. Giving approval or disapproval—implies that the nurse has the right to pass judgment on the "goodness" or "badness" of the client's behavior.
4. Agreeing or disagreeing—implies that the nurse has the right to pass judgment on whether the client's ideas or opinions are "right" or "wrong."
5. Giving advice—implies that the nurse knows what is best for the client, and that the client is incapable of any self-direction.
6. Probing—pushing for answers to issues the client does not wish to discuss, causing the client to feel used and valued only for what is shared with the nurse.
7. Defending (what the client has criticized)—implies that he or she has no right to express ideas, opinions, or feelings.
8. Requesting an explanation—implies that the client must defend his or her behavior or feelings.
9. Belittling feelings expressed—causes the client to feel insignificant or unimportant.
10. Making stereotypical comments (clichés and trite expressions)—is meaningless in a nurse-client relationship.
11. Using denial—blocks discussion with the client and avoids helping the client identify and explore areas of difficulty.
12. Interpreting—results in the therapist telling the client the meaning of his or her experience.
13. Introducing an unrelated topic—causes the nurse to take over the direction of the discussion.
14. Indicating the existence of an external source of power—encourages the client to project blame for his or her thoughts or behaviors on others.

E. Process recordings
1. Process recordings are written reports of verbal interactions with clients and used to improve interpersonal communication techniques.
2. The written record provides a means for the nurse to analyze both the content and the pattern of the interaction.

F. Active listening
1. To listen actively is to be attentive to what the client is saying, both verbally and nonverbally.

2. Several nonverbal behaviors have been designed as facilitative skills for attentive listening. They can be identified by the acronym SOLER.
   a. S—Sit squarely facing the client.
   b. O—Observe an open posture.
   c. L—Lean forward toward the client.
   d. E—Establish eye contact.
   e. R—Relax.
G. Feedback
   1. Feedback is useful when it is conveyed in the following manner:
      a. Descriptive rather than evaluative and focused on the behavior rather than on the client
      b. Specific rather than general
      c. Directed toward behavior that the client has the capacity to modify
      d. Imparting information rather than offering advice
      e. Well-timed
VI. Summary
VII. Review Questions

LEARNING ACTIVITIES

I. Conditions Essential to Development of a Therapeutic Relationship

Situation: Pam comes to the psychiatric clinic for assistance with more adaptive coping. Nurse Jones will be her therapist.

Match the behaviors described on the right with the essential condition for therapeutic relationship development listed on the left.

_____1. Rapport

a. Nurse Jones does not approve of Pam's gay lifestyle but accepts her unconditionally nonetheless.

_____2. Trust

b. Nurse Jones and Pam develop an immediate mutual regard for each other.

_____3. Respect

c. Pam knows that Nurse Jones is always honest with her and will tell her the truth even if it is sometimes painful.

_____4. Genuineness

d. Pam knows that Nurse Jones will not tell anyone else about what they discuss in therapy.

_____5. Empathy

e. When Pam talks about her problems, Nurse Jones listens objectively and encourages Pam to reflect on her feelings about the situation.

II. Phases of Relationship Development

Identify the appropriate phase of relationship development for each of the following tasks. The four phases include:

a. preinteraction phase
b. orientation (introductory) phase
c. working phase
d. termination phase

_____1. Pam and Nurse Jones set goals for their time together.

_____2. Nurse Jones reads Pam's previous medical records.

_____3. Having identified Pam's problem, they discuss aspects for possible change and ways to accomplish them.

_____4. They establish a mutual contract for intervention.

_____5. The established goals have been met.

_____6. Nurse Jones explores her feelings about working with a gay person.

_____7. Pam weighs the benefits and consequences of various alternatives for change.

_____8. Pam and Nurse Jones discuss a plan of action for Pam to employ in the event of stressful situations following therapy.

_____9. Pam cries and says she cannot stop coming to therapy.

_____10. Nurse Jones gives Pam positive feedback for attempting to make adaptive changes in her life.

III. Interpersonal Communication Techniques

After reading the communication on the left, indicate what technique the nurse has used, and whether the technique is therapeutic or nontherapeutic. Selections may be made from the list below. (Client [Ct], Nurse [Ns])

Giving recognition   Indicating an external source of power   Giving advice
Focusing   Voicing doubt   Belittling feelings
Giving reassurance   Exploring   Reflecting
Giving broad openings   Requesting an explanation   Rejecting
Verbalizing the implied   Restating   Defending

1. Ct: "The FBI wants to kill me.
   Ns: "I find that hard to believe." _____ T N

2. Ns Asst: "Mr. J. always calls me sweetie pie. I
            get so angry when he does that."
   Ns: "Perhaps you should consider how *he* is feeling." _____ T N

3. Ct: "My daddy always tucked me into bed at night."
   Ns: "I'd like to talk more about your relationship with
       your father." _____ T N

4. Ns to Ct: "Good morning, Sue. I see you are
            wearing the hair bow you made in OT." _____ T N

5. Ct: "I didn't really mean it when I said I wanted to die."
   Ns: "What makes you say those kinds of things?" _____ T N

6. Ct: "Do you think I should get a divorce?"
   Ns: "What do you think would be best for you?" _____ T N

7. Ct: "Whenever I ask for a different therapy, my doctor
       just ignores me!"
   Ns: "I'm sure he knows what's best for you." _____ T N

8. Ct: "We always had such fun on holidays when I was
       growing up."
   Ns: "Tell me more about what it was like when you
       were a little girl." _____ T N

9. Ct: (Mute. Refusing to talk.)
   Ns: "It must have been a horrible experience for you
       being the only survivor of the automobile accident." _____ T N

10. Ct: "I don't think my life will ever be the same again."
    Ns: "Cheer up. Everything's going to be okay." _____ T N

11. Ct: "I feel like such a failure in the eyes of my family."
    Ns: "You feel as though you have let your family down." _____ T N

12. Ct: "Do you think I should leave home and get an
        apartment of my own?"
    Ns: "I think you would be much better off away from
        your parents." _____ T N

13. Ct: "Good morning, nurse."
    Ns: "Good morning, Patricia. What would you like
        to talk about today?" _____ T N

14. Ct: "I'd like to talk about my relationship with my
        boyfriend, Jack."
    Ns: "Oh, let's don't talk about that. You talk about
        that too much." _____ T N

15. Ct: "I want to call my husband."
    Ns: "Why do you want to talk to him after the way
    he treated you?"   _____ T N

TEST QUESTIONS

1. When there is congruence between what the nurse is feeling and what is being
   expressed, the nurse is conveying:
   a. respect
   - b. genuineness
   c. sympathy
   d. rapport

2. Sally has made the decision to leave her alcoholic husband. She is feeling very
   depressed right now. Which of the following statements by the nurse conveys
   empathy?

   a. "I know you are feeling very depressed right now. I felt the same way when
   I decided to leave my husband. But I can tell you from personal experience,
   you are doing the right thing."
   - b. "I can understand that you are feeling depressed right now. It was a very
   difficult decision to make. I'll sit here with you for a while."

3. Sally has made the decision to leave her alcoholic husband. She is feeling very
   depressed right now. Which of the following statements by the nurse conveys
   sympathy?

   - a. "I know you are feeling very depressed right now. I felt the same way when
   I decided to leave my husband. But I can tell you from personal experience,
   you are doing the right thing."
   b. "I can understand that you are feeling depressed right now. It was a very
   difficult decision to make. I'll sit here with you for a while."

4. Which of the following tasks takes place during the Working Phase of relationship
   development?
   a. Establishing a contract for intervention.
   b. Examining feelings about working with a particular client.
   c. Establishing a plan for continuing aftercare.
   - d. Promoting the client's insight and perception of reality.

Situation: Roy is a client on the psychiatric unit. He has a diagnosis of antisocial personality disorder. Jack is assigned as Roy's nurse.

5. Occasionally, Roy loses his temper and expresses his anger inappropriately. Which of the following statements would be appropriate feedback for Roy's angry outbursts?
   a. "You were very rude to interrupt the group the way you did."
   b. "You accomplish nothing when you lose your temper like that."
   c. "Showing your anger in that manner is very childish and insensitive."
   • d. "You became angry in group, raised your voice, stomped out, and slammed the door."

6. Roy says to Jack, "I don't belong in this place with all these loonies. My doctor must be crazy!" Which of the following responses by Jack is most appropriate?
   • a. "You are here for a psychological evaluation."
   b. "I'm sure your doctor has your best interests in mind."
   c. "Why do you think you don't belong here?"
   d. "Just bide your time. You'll be out of here soon."

7. Nancy, a pregnant adolescent, asks the nurse on the psychiatric unit, "Do you think I should give my baby up for adoption?" Which of the following statements by the nurse is most appropriate?
   a. "It would probably be best for you and the baby."
   b. "Why would you want to give it up for adoption?"
   • c. "What do *you* think would be the best thing for you to do?"
   c. "I'm afraid you would feel very guilty afterward if you gave your baby away."

8. The purpose of providing feedback is to:
   a. Give the client good advice.
   b. Tell the client how to behave.
   c. Evaluate the client's behavior.
   • d. Give the client information.

9. When interviewing a psychiatric client, which of the following nonverbal behaviors should the nurse be careful to avoid?
   a. Maintaining eye contact
   • b. Leaning back with arms crossed
   c. Sitting directly facing the client
   d. Smiling

10. Which of the following suggests the establishment of *rapport*?
    a. The nurse accepts the client even though she does not approve of his behavior.
    b. The client knows that the nurse will not tell others about what they discuss.
  • c. The nurse and client develop a close, mutual regard for each other.
    d. The client knows that the nurse will always tell him the truth, no matter how painful.

CHAPTER 6. THE NURSING PROCESS IN PSYCHIATRIC/ MENTAL HEALTH NURSING

CHAPTER FOCUS

The focus of this chapter is to introduce the reader to each of the six steps of the nursing process and to identify the use of each in psychiatric nursing. Cultural concepts, as they pertain to assessment of psychiatric clients, are discussed. Documentation to the nursing process is described.

LEARNING OBJECTIVES

After reading this chapter, the student will be able to:
1. Define *nursing process*.
2. Identify six steps of the nursing process and describe nursing actions associated with each.
3. Describe the benefits of using nursing diagnoses.
4. Discuss the list of nursing diagnoses approved by the North American Nursing Diagnosis Association for clinical use and testing.
5. Define and differentiate between *culture* and *ethnicity*.
6. Describe six phenomena with which to identify cultural differences.
7. Apply the six steps of the nursing process used in the care of a client within the psychiatric setting.
8. Document client care that validates use of the nursing process.

KEY TERMS

nursing process
nursing diagnosis
interdisciplinary
problem-oriented recording (POR)
Focus Charting®
PIE Charting
stereotyping
acculturation
culture
ethnicity

CHAPTER OUTLINE/LECTURE NOTES

I. Introduction
   A. The **nursing process** provides a systematic framework for the delivery of nursing care.

B. The nursing process fulfills the requirements for a *scientific methodology* in order for nursing to be considered a profession.

II. The Nursing Process
  A. Definition
    1. A six-step, problem-solving approach
    2. Goal-directed, with the objective being delivery of quality client care
    3. Dynamic, not static
  B. Standards of care: The standards of care for psychiatric nursing are written around the six steps of the nursing process:
    1. Standard I. Assessment: The psychiatric/mental health nurse collects client health data.
      a. Sociocultural concepts
        (1) **Culture** describes a particular society's entire way of living, encompassing shared patterns of belief, feeling, and knowledge that guide people's conduct and are passed down from generation to generation.
        (2) **Ethnicity** relates to people who identify with each other because of a shared heritage.
        (3) Nurses must understand these cultural concepts because cultural influences affect human behavior, the interpretation of human behavior, and responses to human behavior.
        (4) Caution must be taken to not assume that all individuals who share a culture or ethnic group are clones. This constitutes **stereotyping**, and must be avoided. All individuals must be appreciated for their uniqueness.
      b. How do cultures differ?
        (1) Communication
          (a) Has its roots in culture.
          (b) Is expressed through language, paralanguage, and gestures.
        (2) Space (the place where the communication occurs)
          (a) Territoriality refers to the innate tendency to own space.
          (b) Density refers to the number of people within a given environmental space.
          (c) Distance is the means by which various cultures use space to communicate.
        (3) Social organization
          (a) Social organizations are the groups within which individuals are acculturated, acquiring knowledge and internalizing values.
          (b) Examples of social organizations are families, religious groups, and ethnic groups.
        (4) Time
          (a) Some cultures place great importance on values that are measured by time, whereas others are actually scornful of clock time.
          (b) Whether individuals perceive time in the present orientation or future orientation influences many aspects of their lives.

(5) Environmental control

    (a) Has to do with the degree to which individuals perceive that they have control over their environment.

    (b) Cultural beliefs and practices influence how individuals respond to their environment during periods of wellness and illness.

(6) Biological variations are differences among people in various racial groups and include body structure, skin color, physiological responses to medication, electrocardiographic patterns, susceptibility to disease, and nutritional preferences and deficiencies.

2. Standard II. Diagnosis: The psychiatric/mental health nurse analyzes the assessment data in determining diagnoses.

  a. Why **nursing diagnosis**?

    (1) Identification and classification of nursing phenomena began in 1973 with the First National Conference on Nursing Diagnosis.

    (2) Both general and specialty standards are written around the six steps of the nursing process, of which nursing diagnosis is an inherent part.

    (3) Diagnosis is defined in most state nursing practice acts as a legal responsibility of nursing.

    (4) Diagnosis promotes autonomy in nursing.

3. Standard III. Outcome identification: The psychiatric/mental health nurse identifies expected outcomes individualized to the client.

  a. Expected outcomes are derived from the diagnosis.

  b. Outcomes must be measurable and estimate a time for attainment.

  c. Outcomes must be realistic for the client's capabilities, and are most effective when formulated by the **interdisciplinary** members, the client, and significant others together.

4. Standard IV. Planning: The psychiatric/mental health nurse develops a plan of care that prescribes interventions to attain expected outcomes.

  a. The care plan is individualized to the client's mental health problems, condition, or needs and is developed in collaboration with the client, significant others, and interdisciplinary team members, if possible.

  b. For each diagnosis identified, the most appropriate interventions, based on current psychiatric/mental health nursing practice and research, are selected.

5. Standard V. Implementation: The psychiatric/mental health nurse implements the interventions identified in the plan of care.

  a. Interventions selected during the planning stage are executed, taking into consideration the nurse's level of practice, education, and certification.

  b. Several specific interventions are included among the standards of psychiatric/mental health clinical nursing practice.

    (1) Standard Va. Counseling. The nurse uses counseling interventions to assist clients in improving or regaining their previous coping abilities, fostering mental health, and preventing mental illness and disability.

 (2) Standard Vb. Milieu Therapy. The nurse provides, structures, and maintains a therapeutic environment in collaboration with the client and other health care providers.

 (3) Standard Vc. Self-care activities. The nurse structures interventions around the client's activities of daily living (ADLs) to foster self-care and mental and physical well-being.

 (4) Standard Vd. Psychobiological interventions. The nurse uses knowledge of psychobiological interventions and applies clinical skills to restore the client's health and prevent further disability.

 (5) Standard Ve. Health teaching. The nurse, through health teaching, assists clients in achieving satisfying, productive, and healthy patterns of living.

 (6) Standard Vf. Case management. The nurse provides case management to coordinate comprehensive health services and ensure continuity of care.

 (7) Standard Vg. Health promotion and health maintenance. The nurse employs strategies and interventions to promote and maintain mental health and prevent mental illness.

 (8) Standards specific to the Advanced Practice Psychiatric-Mental Health Nurse:

  (i) Standard Vh. Psychotherapy. The Advanced Practice Psychiatric-Mental Health Nurse uses individual, group, and family psychotherapy, and other therapeutic treatments to assist clients in preventing mental illness and disability, treating mental health disorders, and improving mental health status and functional abilities.

  (ii) Standard Vi. Prescriptive authority and treatment. The Advanced Practice Psychiatric-Mental Health Nurse uses prescriptive authority, procedures, and treatments in accordance with state and federal laws and regulations, to treat symptoms of psychiatric illness and improve functional health status.

  (iii)Standard Vj. Consultation. The Advanced Practice Psychiatric-Mental Health Nurse provides consultation to enhance the abilities of other clinicians to provide services for clients and effect change in the system.

6. Standard VI. Evaluation: The psychiatric/mental health nurse evaluates the client's progress in attaining expected outcomes.

 a. The nurse measures the success of the interventions in meeting the outcome criteria.

 b. Nursing diagnoses, outcomes, and plan of care are reviewed and revised as need is determined.

 c. Client's response to treatment is documented, validating use of the nursing process in the delivery of care.

III. Applying the Nursing Process in the Psychiatric Setting

 A. Role of the nurse in psychiatry

1. To assist the client to successfully adapt to stressors within the environment.
2. Goals are directed toward change in thoughts, feelings, and behaviors that are age-appropriate and congruent with local and cultural norms.
3. Nursing is a valuable member of the interdisciplinary team, providing a service that is unique and based on sound knowledge of psychopathology, scope of practice, and legal implications of the role.

IV. Documentation to the Nursing Process
    A. Documentation of the steps of the nursing is often considered as evidence in determining certain cases of negligence by nurses.
    B. Also required by some health care organization accrediting associations.
    C. Examples of documentation that reflect use of the nursing process are as follows:
        1. **Problem-Oriented Recording (POR)**
           a. Has a list of problems as its basis
           b. Uses subjective, objective, assessment, plan, intervention, and evaluation (SOAPIE)
        2. **Focus Charting®**
           a. The main perspective is to choose a "focus" for documentation. A focus may be:
              (1) a nursing diagnosis.
              (2) a current client concern or behavior.
              (3) a significant change in the client's status or behavior.
              (4) a significant event in the client's therapy.
           b. The focus cannot be a medical diagnosis.
           c. Focus charting uses a data, action, and response (DAR) format.
        3. The "A PIE" Method
           a. A problem-oriented system
           b. Utilizes flow sheets as accompanying documentation
           c. Uses an assessment, problem, intervention, and evaluation (A PIE) format
V. Summary
VI. Review Questions

LEARNING ACTIVITY

The Nursing Process: A Case Study

Read the following case study and follow the directions given below for application of the nursing process.

Situation: Sam is presented through the emergency department to the psychiatric unit of a major medical center. He was taken to the hospital by local police, who were called by department store security when Sam frightened shoppers by yelling loudly to "imaginary" people and threatening to harm anyone who came close to him.

On the psychiatric unit, Sam keeps to himself, and walks away when anyone who approaches him. He talks and laughs to himself, and tilts his head to the side, as if listening. When the nurse attempts to talk to him, he shouts, "Get away from me. I know you are one of them!" He picks up a chair, as if to use it for protection.

Sam's appearance is unkempt. His clothes are dirty and wrinkled, his hair is oily and uncombed, and there is an obvious body odor about him. The physician admits Sam with a diagnosis of paranoid schizophrenia, and orders chlorpromazine (Thorazine) and benztropine (Cogentin) on both a scheduled and p.r.n. basis.

1. Identify four segments of information from the assessment data that would be significant to nursing.

    a. _____
    b. _____
    c. _____
    d. _____

2. List appropriate nursing diagnoses from analysis of the data described in question 1.

    a. _____
    b. _____
    c. _____
    d. _____

3. Provide outcome criteria for the four nursing diagnoses.

    a. _____
    b. _____
    c. _____
    d. _____

4. Select appropriate nursing interventions to achieve the outcome criteria.

TEST QUESTIONS

Six cultural phenomena have been identified that vary among cultural groups and affect health care. Match the situations on the right to the six phenomena on the left.

___d___ 1. Communication

a. Tony, a Mexican American, refuses to go to the clinic for his check-up. He feels very uncomfortable when the Physician's Assistant stands so close to him and touches him.

<u> a </u> 2. Space

b. When Andy, an African American, complains to the physician of weakness and joint pain, the physician suspects sickle cell anemia.

<u> c </u> 3. Social Organization

c. Antoinette, an Italian American, expects to have her husband, parents, siblings, in-laws, and various other relatives present when she gives birth to her first child.

<u> e </u> 4. Time

d. Upon admission to the hospital, Coni Li, an Asian American, explained to the dietitian her preferences for foods that subscribe to *yin* and *yang*. She became very upset when she learned that the dietitian had no knowledge of the concept of *yin* and *yang*.

<u> f </u> 5. Environmental Control

e. Jose, a Latino American, does not believe that he needs to go to the doctor unless he is ill. He does not get routine check-ups, even though his company would pay for them.

<u> b </u> 6. Biological variations

f. Josie, a Native American, prefers to see her *shaman* (her religious healer) for health care than the physician at the community clinic.

7. Laura is a nurse on an inpatient psychiatric unit. Much of her time is spent observing client activity, talking with clients, and striving to maintain a therapeutic environment in collaboration with other health care providers. This specific example of the implementation step of the nursing process is called:
   a. health teaching
   b. case management
 • c. milieu therapy
   d. self-care activities

8. Which of the following statements about nursing diagnosis is true?
   a. Nursing diagnosis is a brand new concept.
   b. All nurses are required by law to write nursing diagnoses.
   c. All nursing diagnoses must be approved by NANDA.

- d. Nursing diagnoses are client responses to actual/potential health problems.

9. Which of the following statements is *not* true about outcomes?
   - a. Expected outcomes are specifically formulated by the nurse.
   - b. Expected outcomes are derived from the nursing diagnosis.
   - c. Expected outcomes must be measurable and estimate a time for attainment.
   - d. Expected outcomes must be realistic for the client's capabilities.

10. Nursing diagnoses are prioritized:
   - a. according to the established goal of care.
   - b. according to life-threatening potential.
   - c. according to the nurse's priority of care.
   - d. according to specific focus of problem resolution.

CHAPTER 7. MILIEU—THE THERAPEUTIC ENVIRONMENT

CHAPTER FOCUS

The focus of this chapter is to introduce the student to the concept of milieu therapy. The role of the nurse in this therapeutic setting is emphasized.

LEARNING OBJECTIVES

After reading this chapter, the student will be able to:
1. Define *milieu therapy.*
2. Explain the goal of therapeutic community/milieu therapy.
3. Identify seven basic assumptions of a therapeutic community.
4. Discuss conditions that characterize a therapeutic community.
5. Identify the various therapies that may be included within the program of therapeutic community, and the health-care workers that make up the interdisciplinary treatment team.
6. Describe the role of the nurse on the interdisciplinary treatment team.

KEY TERMS

milieu
milieu therapy

CHAPTER OUTLINE/LECTURE NOTES

I.   Introduction
   A. Standard Vb of the ANA Standards of Psychiatric-Mental Health Nursing Practice states, "The psychiatric-mental health nurse provides, structures, and maintains a therapeutic environment in collaboration with the client and other health-care providers."
II. **Milieu**, Defined
   A. **Milieu therapy** or therapeutic community is defined as a scientific structuring of the environment in order to effect behavioral changes and to improve the psychological health and functioning of the individual.
   B. Within the therapeutic-community setting the client is expected to learn adaptive coping, interaction, and relationship skills that can be generalized to other aspects of his or her life.
III. Basic Assumptions
   A. The health of each individual is to be realized and encouraged to grow.
   B. Every interaction is an opportunity for therapeutic intervention.
   C. The client owns his or her own environment.
   D. Each client owns his or her own behavior.
   E. Peer pressure is a useful and powerful tool.

F. Inappropriate behaviors are dealt with as they occur.

G. Restrictions and punishment are to be avoided.

IV. Conditions That Promote a Therapeutic Community

    A. Basic physiological needs are fulfilled.

    B. The physical facilities are conducive to achievement of the goals of therapy.

    C. A democratic form of self-government exists.

    D. Unit responsibilities are assigned according to client capabilities.

    E. A structured program of social and work-related activities is scheduled as part of the treatment program.

    F. Community and family are included in the program of therapy in an effort to facilitate discharge from the hospital.

V. The Program of Therapeutic Community

    A. The program is directed by an interdisciplinary team.

    B. A treatment plan is formulated by the team.

    C. All disciplines sign the treatment plan and meet weekly to update the plan as needed.

    D. Disciplines may include psychiatry, psychology, nursing, social work, occupational therapy, recreational therapy, art therapy, music therapy, dietetics, and chaplain's service.

VI. Role of the Nurse

    A. Through use of the nursing process, nurses manage the therapeutic environment on a 24-hour basis.

    B. Nurses have the responsibility for ensuring that clients' physiological and psychological needs are met.

    C. Nurses also are responsible for:

        1. Medication administration.

        2. Development of a one-to-one relationship.

        3. Setting limits on unacceptable behavior.

        4. Client education.

VI. Summary

VII. Review Questions

LEARNING ACTIVITIES

I. The Interdisciplinary Team

Identify the appropriate member of the interdisciplinary team for the activity listed. Choices may be made from the following list:

psychiatrist	psychiatric staff nurse	art therapist
clinical psychologist	occupational therapist	dietitian
mental health technician	psychodramatist	chaplain
psychiatric social worker	recreational therapist	music therapist
psychiatric clinical nurse specialist		

1. Accompanies clients to see a movie. _____

2. Helps clients identify unconscious
   feelings through their drawings. _____

3. Conducts psychological testing to assist
   the psychiatrist determine a correct diagnosis. _____

4. Serves the spiritual needs of psychiatric clients. _____

5. Monitors nutritional needs for client with
   special requirements. _____

6. Teaches relaxation techniques through
   the use of music. _____

7. Conducts assertiveness training. _____

8. Prescribes electroconvulsive therapy for
   a depressed client. _____

9. Administers medication. _____

10. Locates appropriate placement for the
    client following hospital discharge. _____

11. Assists clients to increase self-esteem by
    providing small craft items for completion
    and display. _____

12. Assists a group of clients to perform in a
    safe environment a situation that otherwise
    would be too painful in real life. _____

13. Works one-to-one with clients and assists the
    psychiatric nurse in running the day-to-day
    activities of the milieu unit. _____

II. The Seven Basic Assumptions of a Therapeutic Community

There are seven basic assumptions upon which a therapeutic community is based. Identify the assumption (from the column on the right) that is the foundation for each of the situations listed on the left.

_____ 1. John came into the TV room and changed the channel in the middle of a program that several others were watching. The group reprimanded him loudly, and returned the TV to the channel they had been watching. They told him they would not tolerate that kind of behavior.

a. The health in each individual is to be realized and encouraged to grow.

_____ 2. Even though she seemed unable to change, Nancy had a great deal of insight into her own behavior. She knew it was maladaptive and she knew it had psychological implications. The nurse focused on Nancy's insight and knowledge to help her find more adaptive ways of coping.

b. Every interaction is an opportunity for therapeutic intervention.

_____ 3. George always started an argument in group therapy. Each time, the group calmed him down with their discussion. When he became violent, however, he was placed in isolation for the safety of himself and others.

c. The client owns his/her own environment.

_____ 4. Fred becomes angry whenever anyone in the group disagrees with him. Members of the group examine Fred's defensiveness, and help him to see how he is coming across to others. They help him to practice more appropriate ways of responding.

d. Each client owns his or her behavior.

_____ 5. Lloyd had always been unable to interact on a personal level with other people. In the milieu environment, he learned new communication skills and had the opportunity to practice relationship development that helped him when he left the hospital.

e. Peer pressure is a useful and powerful tool.

_____ 6. Kevin told the nurse of being arrested for driving the getaway car in an armed robbery. He stated, "I don't know why they grabbed me. Jack did the stealing! He made me drive the car." The nurse responded, "Kevin, no one made you drive the car. You made that choice yourself. Now you must own up to that decision."

f. Inappropriate behavior is dealt with as it occurs.

_____ 7. Carol was elected unit president at the community meeting. She assigns chores for the week, and calls for a vote concerning late privileges for clients on Saturday night.

g. Restrictions and punishment are to be avoided.

TEST QUESTIONS

1. Which of the following statements is true about milieu therapy?
    a. Punishments are used to eliminate negative behaviors.
    b. Interpersonal therapy is the foundation for the program of treatment.
    c. The staff performs all activities of care for the clients.
  • d. The environment is structured so that stresses are used as opportunities for learning.

2. To reinforce the democratic form of self-government on a milieu unit:

a. Clients are allowed to set forth the type of punishment for a peer who violates the rules.
b. Clients may choose whether or not to attend daily community meetings.
- c. Clients participate in decision making that affects management of the unit.
d. Professional staff do not attend community meetings.

3. Jack is a client on the psychiatric unit. Jack expressed at community meeting which movie he wanted to see that night. His choice was denied because of the majority rule. At movie time that evening, Jack put the tape he wanted to view into the VCR. He was reprimanded by his peers, who removed the tape and put in the one voted on by the majority. This is an example of which basic assumption of milieu therapy?
a. Every interaction is an opportunity for therapeutic intervention.
- b. Peer pressure is a useful and powerful tool.
c. Restrictions and punishment are to be avoided.
d. The client owns his/her own environment.

4. Jack's physician decides to have Jack undergo psychological testing. Which of the following members of the interdisciplinary team would Jack's physician consult for this purpose?
a. The occupational therapist.
b. The psychiatric social worker.
- c. The clinical psychologist.
d. The clinical nurse specialist.

5. Which of the following best describes the role of the nurse in the therapeutic milieu of a psychiatric unit?
- a. The member of the treatment team who is responsible for management of the therapeutic milieu.
b. A member of the treatment team who develops the medical diagnosis for all clients on the unit.
c. The team member who provides for the spiritual and comfort needs of the client and his or her family.
d. The team member who conducts individual, group, and family therapy after an in-depth psychosocial history.

CHAPTER 8. INTERVENTION IN GROUPS

CHAPTER FOCUS

The focus of this chapter is on the dynamics and functions of therapeutic groups. The role of the nurse in this type of intervention is explored.

LEARNING OBJECTIVES

After reading this chapter, the student will be able to:
1. Define a *group*.
2. Discuss eight functions of a group.
3. Identify various types of groups.
4. Describe physical conditions that influence groups.
5. Discuss "curative factors" that occur in groups.
6. Describe the phases of group development.
7. Identify various leadership styles in groups.
8. Identify various roles that members assume within a group.
9. Discuss psychodrama and family therapy as specialized forms of group therapy.
10. Describe the role of the nurse in group therapy.

KEY TERMS

altruism
autocratic
catharsis
democratic
group therapy
laissez-faire
psychodrama
family therapy
universality
genogram
therapeutic group

CHAPTER OUTLINE/LECTURE NOTES

I. Introduction
   A. Health-care professionals not only share their personal lives with groups of people but also encounter multiple group situations in their professional operations.
   B. Clients learn from each other in a group setting.
II. The group is a collection of individuals whose association is founded on shared commonalities of interest, values, norms, or purpose.
III. Functions of a Group

Copyright © 2002, F. A. Davis Company

A. Socialization—the teaching of social norms.

B. Support—fellow members are available in time of need.

C. Task completion—assistance is provided when completion is enhanced by group involvement.

D. Camaraderie—individuals receive joy and pleasure from interactions with significant others.

E. Informational—learning takes place when group members share their knowledge with the others in the group.

F. Normative—different groups enforce the established norms in various ways.

G. Empowerment—change can be effected by groups at times when individuals alone are ineffective.

H. Governance—large organizations often have leadership that is provided by groups rather than a single individual.

IV. Types of Groups

A. Task groups—are formed to accomplish a specific outcome.

B. Teaching groups—focus on conveying knowledge and information to a number of individuals.

C. Supportive or **therapeutic groups**—are concerned with preventing possible future upsets by educating the participants in effective ways of dealing with emotional stress arising from situational or developmental crises.

1. Therapeutic groups versus **group therapy**

    a. Group therapy has a sound theoretical base and their leaders generally have advanced degrees in psychology, social work, nursing, or medicine.

    b. To a lesser degree, therapeutic groups are based in theory. Focus is on group relations, interactions between group members, and the consideration of a selected issue.

    c. Leaders of both types of groups must be knowledgeable about group *process* (the way in which group members interact with each other), as well as group *content* (the topic or issue being discussed in the group).

D. Self-help groups—are composed of individuals with a similar problem. These groups serve to reduce the possibilities of further emotional distress, which may lead to pathology and necessary treatment. They may or may not have a professional leader; they may be run by members, and leadership often rotates from member to member.

V. Physical Conditions

A. Seating. It is best when there is no barrier between the members. For example, a circle of chairs is better than chairs set around a table.

B. Size. Size of the group makes a difference in the interaction among members. Seven or eight members provide a favorable climate for optimal group interaction and relationship development.

C. Membership. Two types of groups exist: *open-ended groups* (those in which members leave and others join at any time during the existence of the group) and *closed-ended groups* (those in which all members join at the time the group is organized and terminate at the end of the designated length of time).

VI. Curative Factors

A. The instillation of hope. By observing the progress of others in the group with similar problems, a group member garners hope that his or her problems can also be resolved.

B. **Universality**. Individuals come to realize that they are not alone in the problems, thoughts, and feelings they are experiencing.

C. The imparting of information. Group members share their knowledge with each other. Leaders of teaching groups also provide information to group members.

D. **Altruism**. Individuals provide assistance and support to each other, thereby creating a positive self-image and promoting self-growth.

E. The corrective recapitulation of the primary family group. Group members are able to re-experience early family conflicts that remain unresolved.

F. The development of socializing techniques. Through interaction with and feedback from other members within the group, individuals are able to correct maladaptive social behaviors and learn and develop new social skills.

G. Imitative behavior. Group members who have mastered a particular psychosocial skill or developmental task serve as valuable role models for others.

H. Interpersonal learning. The group offers many and varied opportunities for interacting with other people.

I. Group cohesiveness. Members develop a sense of belonging that separates the individual ("I am") from the group ("we are").

J. **Catharsis**. Within the group, members are able to express both positive and negative feelings.

K. Existential factors. The group is able to assist individual members to take direction of their own lives and to accept responsibility for the quality of their existence.

VII. Phases of Group Development

  A. Initial or orientation phase

    1. Leader and members work together to establish rules and goals for the group.

    2. The leader promotes trust and ensures that the rules do not interfere with the fulfillment of the goals.

    3. Members are superficial and overly polite. Trust has not yet been established.

  B. Middle or working phase

    1. Productive work toward completion of the task is undertaken.

    2. Leader role diminishes and becomes one of facilitator.

    3. Trust has been established between the members and cohesiveness exists. Conflict is managed by the group members themselves.

  C. Final or termination phase

    1. A sense of loss, precipitating the grief process, may be experienced by group members.

    2. The leader encourages the group members to discuss these feelings of loss, and to reminisce about the accomplishments of the group.

    3. Feelings of abandonment may be experienced by some members. Grief for previous losses may be triggered.

VIII. Leadership Styles

A. **Autocratic**. The focus is on the leader, on whom the members are dependent for problem solving, decision making, and permission to perform. Production is high, but morale is low.

B. **Democratic**. The focus is on the members, who are encouraged to participate fully in problem solving of issues that relate to the group, including taking action to effect change. Production is somewhat lower than it is with autocratic leadership, but morale is much higher.

C. **Laissez-faire**. There is no focus in this type of leadership. Goals are undefined, and members do as they please. Productivity and morale are very low.

IX. Member Roles: Members play one of three types of roles within a group.

A. Task roles. Roles that serve to complete the task of the group.

B. Maintenance roles. Roles that serve to maintain or enhance group processes.

C. Individual (personal) roles. Roles that serve to fulfill personal or individual needs.

IX. **Psychodrama**

A. Defined as a type of group therapy that employs a dramatic approach in which clients become "actors" in life situation scenarios.

B. An identified client (called the protagonist) is selected to portray a life situation. Other members of the group play the roles of people with whom the protagonist has unresolved issues. Group members who do not participate in the drama act as the audience, and the group leader is called the director.

C. The purpose is to provide the client with a safe place in which to confront unresolved conflicts and hopefully progress toward resolution.

D. Nurses who work as psychodramatists require specialist training beyond the master's degree.

X. The Family as a Group

A. **Family therapy** is defined as an attempt to modify the relationships in a family to achieve harmony.

B. The family is viewed as a system in which the members are interdependent, and a change in one part (member) affects or creates change in all the other parts (members). Focus is on the family, rather than on the individual.

C. Family members establish goals for change with guidance from the therapist. Change occurs through open, honest communication among all family members.

D. Some therapists use **genograms** to enhance their understanding of the dynamics within a family.

E. Most nurses who conduct family therapy have advanced degrees with considerable knowledge about family theory.

F. Staff nurses should have a basic understanding of family dynamics and the ability to distinguish between functional and dysfunctional behaviors within a family system.

XI. The Role of the Nurse in Group Therapy

A. Nurses who work in psychiatry may lead various types of therapeutic groups, such as client education groups, assertiveness training, support groups for clients with similar problems, parent groups, transition to discharge groups, and others.

B. Guidelines set forth by the American Nurses' Association specify that nurses who serve as group psychotherapists should have a minimum of a master's degree in psychiatric nursing.

XIII. Summary

XIV. Review Questions

LEARNING ACTIVITIES

Allow students to use clinical time to attend various types of groups. Following attendance, students should report back to the clinical group in terms of the following:

1. Type of group attended (task, teaching, supportive/therapeutic, self-help)
2. Type of leadership identified for the group (give rationale for determination)
3. Member roles identified (task roles, maintenance roles, personal roles)
4. Description of group dynamics

Suggestions for possible group attendance include the following:

1. Task groups:
    a. Various hospital committees
    b. Interdisciplinary treatment team meetings
    c. Nursing faculty curriculum committee meeting
    d. Discharge planning meetings

2. Teaching groups:
    a. Prepared childbirth classes
    b. Diabetes education classes
    c. Daily living skills groups
    d. Medication classes
    e. Transition to discharge groups

3. Supportive or therapeutic groups:
    a. Assertiveness training groups
    b. Survivors groups (e.g., victims of sexual abuse)
    c. Self-awareness groups
    d. Bereavement groups
    e. Groups for individuals coping with cancer

4. Self-help groups:
    a. Alcoholics Anonymous
    b. Al-Anon
    c. Parents without Partners
    d. Weight Watchers
    e. Overeaters Anonymous
    f. Gamblers Anonymous
    g. Narcotics Anonymous

TEST QUESTIONS

1. Jane, a psychiatric nurse, leads a supportive-therapeutic group on the psychiatric unit. It is an open group, and clients come and go within the group as they are admitted to and discharged from the unit. Members discuss unresolved issues and ways to cope with stress in their lives. One evening when the group was breaking up, Jane heard one client say to another, "I never thought that other people had the same problems that I have." This statement represents which of Yalom's curative factors?
    a. Catharsis
    b. Group cohesiveness
  • c. Universality
    d. Imitative behavior

2. Meredith has been in the group for 2 weeks now. She dominates the conversation and doesn't permit others to participate. Meredith is assuming which of the following roles within the group?
    a. Aggressor
    b. Dominator
    c. Recognition Seeker
  • d. Monopolizer

3. One evening, several of the group members spoke up in group and expressed their dissatisfaction with Meredith's behavior in the group. They encouraged others in the group to express their feelings as well. Together they decided that from then on all members who wished to do so would get a turn to talk in group, and time would be monitored so that everyone would get their turn. Jane remained silent during this group interaction. Which type of leadership style does Jane demonstrate?
    a. Autocratic
    b. Democratic
  • c. Laissez-faire

4. Although Meredith talks a lot in group, Jane notices that much of her expressions are kept on the superficial level. Jane decides that Meredith might benefit from psychodrama. She makes a referral for Meredith to the psychodramatist. Which of the following statements is *not* true about psychodrama?
    a. It provides a safe setting in which to discuss painful issues.
    b. Peers will act out roles that represent individuals with whom Meredith has unresolved conflicts.

- c. Meredith can choose who will play the role of *her*, while she observe the interaction from the audience.
  d. After the drama has been completed, a discussion will be held with members of the audience.

5. Michael, an RN with 3 years' experience on a psychiatric inpatient unit, has taken a position in a day treatment program where he will be leading some groups. Which of the following groups is Michael qualified to lead?
   - a. A parenting group
   b. A psychotherapy group
   c. A psychodrama group
   d. A family therapy group

Match the individual on the right to the role he or she is playing within the group.

6. e___Aggressor

7. h___Blocker

8. f___Dominator

9. d___Help seeker

10. a___Monopolizer

11. c___Mute or silent member

a. Nancy talks incessantly in group. When someone else tries to make a comment, she refuses to allow them to speak.

b. On the first day the group meets, Valarie shares the intimate details of her incestual relationship with her father.

c. Colleen listens with interest to everything the other members say, but she does not say anything herself in group.

d. Violet is obsessed with her physical appearance. Although she is beautiful, she has little self-confidence and needs continuous positive feedback. She states, "Maybe if I became a blond my boyfriend would love me more."

e. Larry states to Violet, "Listen, dummy, you need more than blond hair to keep the guy around. A bit more in the brains department would help!"

f. At the beginning of the group meeting, Dan says, "All right now, I have a date tonight. I want this meeting over on time! I'll keep track of the time and let everyone know when their time is up. When I say you're done, you're done, understand?"

12, __g__ Recognition seeker

g. Joyce says, "I won my first beauty contest when I was 6 months old. Can you imagine? And I've been winning them ever since. I was prom queen when I was 16, Miss Rose Petal when I was 19, Miss Silver City at 21. And next I go to the state contest. It's just all so exciting!"

13. __b__ Seducer

h. Joe, an RN on the care planning committee says, "What a stupid suggestion. Nursing Diagnosis?! I won't even discuss the matter. We have been doing our care plans this way for 20 years. I refuse to even consider changing."

CHAPTER 9. INTERVENING IN CRISES

CHAPTER FOCUS

The focus of this chapter is to introduce the student to the concept of crisis and the therapy of crisis intervention. The role of the nurse in crisis intervention is emphasized.

LEARNING OBJECTIVES

After reading this chapter, the student will be able to:
1. Define *crisis*.
2. Describe four phases in the development of a crisis.
3. Identify types of crises that occur in people's lives.
4. Discuss the goal of crisis intervention.
5. Describe the steps in crisis intervention.
6. Identify the role of the nurse in crisis intervention.
7. Apply the nursing process to clients experiencing crises.
8. Apply the nursing process to clients expressing anger or aggression.

KEY TERMS

crisis
crisis intervention

CHAPTER OUTLINE/LECTURE NOTES

I. Introduction
   A. Any stressful situation can precipitate a **crisis**.
   B. Assistance with problem solving during the crisis period preserves self-esteem and promotes growth with resolution.
II. Crisis, Defined
   A. Crisis has been defined as a psychological disequilibrium in a person who confronts a hazardous circumstance that, for that person, constitutes an important problem that can, for the time being, neither be escaped nor solved with his or her customary problem-solving resources.
   B. Assumptions on which the concept of crisis is based
      1. Crisis occurs in all individuals at one time or another and is not necessarily equated with psychopathology.
      2. Crises are precipitated by specific identifiable events.
      3. Crises are personal by nature.
      4. Crises are acute, not chronic, and will be resolved in one way or another within a brief period.
      5. A crisis situation contains the potential for psychological growth or deterioration.

III. Phases in the Development of a Crisis
   A. The individual is exposed to a precipitating stressor.
   B. When previous problem-solving techniques do not relieve the stressor, anxiety increases further.
   C. All possible resources, both internal and external, are called on to resolve the problem and relieve the discomfort.
   D. If resolution does not occur in previous phases, the tension mounts beyond a further threshold or its burden increases over time to a breaking point. Major disorganization of the individual with drastic results often occurs.
IV. Types of Crises
   A. Dispositional crises are acute responses to external situational stressors.
   B. Crises of anticipated life transitions occur with normal life-cycle transitions that may be anticipated but over which the individual may feel a lack of control.
   C. Crises resulting from traumatic stress are those that are precipitated by an unexpected, external stressor over which the individual has little or no control and by which he or she feels emotionally overwhelmed and defeated.
   D. Maturational or developmental crises occur in response to situations that trigger emotions related to unresolved conflicts in one's life.
   E. A crisis reflecting psychopathology is one in which preexisting psychopathology has been instrumental in precipitating the crisis or in which psychopathology significantly impairs or complicates adaptive resolution of the crisis.
   F. Psychiatric emergencies are crisis situations in which general functioning has been severely impaired and the individual has been rendered incompetent or unable to assume personal responsibility.
V. **Crisis Intervention**
   A. The minimum therapeutic goal of crisis intervention is psychological resolution of the individual's immediate crisis and restoration to at least the level of functioning that existed before the crisis period.
   B. A maximum goal is improvement in functioning above the precrisis level.
   C. The crisis usually lasts from 4 to 6 weeks.
VI. Phases of Crisis Intervention: The Role of the Nurse
   A. Nurses may be called on to function as crisis helpers in virtually any setting committed to the practice of nursing.
      1. Phase 1. Assessment. Information is gathered regarding the precipitating stressor and the resulting crisis that prompted the individual to seek professional help.
      2. Phase 2. Planning of Therapeutic Intervention. From the assessment data, the nurse selects appropriate nursing diagnoses that reflect the immediacy of the crisis situation. Desired outcome criteria are established. Appropriate nursing actions are selected taking into consideration the type of crisis, as well as the individual's strengths and available resources for support.
      3. Phase 3. Intervention. The actions identified in the planning phase are implemented. A reality-oriented approach is used. A rapid working relationship is established by showing unconditional acceptance, by active

listening, and by attending to immediate needs. A problem-solving model becomes the basis for change.

    4. Phase 4. Evaluation of Crisis Resolution and Anticipatory Planning. A reassessment is conducted to determine if the stated objectives were achieved. A plan of action is developed for the individual to deal with the stressor should it recur.

VII. Crisis on the Inpatient Unit: Anger/Aggression Management

  A. Assessment

    1. Anger

      a. A number of characteristics describe anger, including frowning, gritting of the teeth, pacing, clenched fists, increased energy, fatigue, withdrawal, flushed face, emotional overcontrol, and change in tone of voice.

      b. Anger is a stage of the grieving process.

      c. Anger turned inward results in depression.

      d. Some individuals need assistance to recognize their true feelings as anger.

    2. Aggression

      a. Aggression can arise from such feeling states as anger, anxiety, tension, guilt, frustration, or hostility.

      b. Aggressive behaviors may be mild, moderate, severe, or extreme.

      c. Aggression may be characterized by sarcasm, verbal or physical threats, degrading comments, throwing or striking objects or people, suicidal or homicidal ideation, self-mutilation, disturbed thought process and perception, and anger disproportionate to an event.

    3. Assessing risk factors

      a. Prevention is the key issue in the management of aggressive or violent behavior.

      b. The violent individual usually feels underlying helplessness.

      c. The most widely recognized risk factor for violence in a treatment setting is a history of assault.

      d. Diagnoses that have the highest association with violent behavior include substance abuse/intoxication, schizophrenia, posttraumatic stress disorder, organic brain disorders, epilepsy, and temporal lobe abnormalities.

      e. The "preassaultive tension state" describes a set of behaviors that are predictive of impending violence.

  B. Diagnosis/outcome identification

    1. Dysfunctional grieving may be used when anger is expressed inappropriately and the etiology is related to a loss.

    2. Ineffective individual coping.

    3. Risk for violence: self-directed or other-directed.

    4. Outcomes evaluate success of the individual in maintaining anger at a manageable level and the prevention of harm to self or others.

  C. Planning/implementation

  D. Evaluation

VIII. Summary

IX. Review Questions

LEARNING ACTIVITIES

I. Types of Crises

Match the situation on the left with the type of crisis listed on the right.

_____ 1. Twenty-four-year-old Harriet was informed that her husband was killed in an industrial accident at the plant where he works. An hour later, she was found walking down a busy highway saying, "I'm looking for my lucky rabbit's foot. Everything will be okay if I can just find my lucky rabbit's foot."

a. Dispositional crisis

_____ 2. Ted was transferred on his job to a distant city. His wife, Jane, had never lived away from her family before. She became despondent, living only for daily phone calls to her relatives back in their home town.

b. Crisis of anticipated life transition

_____ 3. Carrie knew when she married Matt that he had a drinking problem, but she believed he would change. Last night, after becoming intoxicated, Matt beat Carrie into unconsciousness. When she regained consciousness, he was gone. She took a taxi to the emergency department of the local hospital.

c. Crisis resulting from traumatic stress

_____ 4. Linda had a history of obsessive-compulsive disorder. She was phobic about germs, and washed her hands many times every day. Last night, after a party, she had sex with a fellow college student she barely knew. Today, she is extremely anxious, and keeps repeating that she knows she has AIDS. Her roommate cannot get her to come out of the shower.

d. Maturational or developmental crisis

_____ 5. At age 13, Sue was raped by her uncle. The abuse continued for several years. He threatened to kill her mother if she told. Sue is 23 years old now, and recently became engaged. She has never had an intimate relationship, and experiences panic attacks at the thought of her wedding night.

e. Crisis reflecting psychopathology

_____ 6. Frank was very proud of his home. He had saved for many years to build it and had virtually built it from the ground up by himself. Last night, while he and his wife were visiting in a nearby town, a tornado ripped through his neighborhood and totally destroyed his home. Frank is devastated, and for more than a week has sat and stared into space, barely eating and rarely speaking.

f. Psychiatric emergency

II. Crisis Intervention: Problem-Solving Process

You are a nurse in the mental health clinic in the town to which Ted and Jane (Situation #2 in the previous activity) have moved. Ted brings Jane to your clinic and explains that she has become nonfunctional since their move. Use the steps of the problem-solving process with the objective of assisting Jane to overcome her despondency.

1. Confront the problem.
2. Identify realistic changes.
3. Explore coping strategies for aspects about her situation that cannot be changed.
4. Identify various alternatives for coping with the situation.
5. Weigh the benefits and consequences of each alternative.
6. Select the most appropriate alternative.

TEST QUESTIONS

Situation: On Thursday, Camille, a college junior, is accompanied to the Student Health Center by her roommate, Nancy. Nancy explains to the nurse that for 3 days Camille has been unable to attend her classes, has cried constantly, and has become panicky whenever Nancy leaves to go to classes and meals. The nurse performs an assessment and finds that Camille does not know the date and has difficulty with short-term memory. Nancy is not aware that Camille has received any bad news recently but offers that Camille is a good student and has been spending long hours at the computer center for nearly 2 weeks working on a major class project, usually returning to the dorm after Nancy is asleep. This is the strategy she has successfully used when working on projects in the past and was the strategy employed through Monday of this week.

1. What crucial information is missing that will *most* assist the nurse to plan interventions that will be helpful for Camille?
    - • a. The precipitating stressor
      b. Camille's usual ability to cope with stress
      c. How far away Camille's home and parents are
      d. The due date of Camille's project

2. Based on the correct answer to question 1, which of the following types of crises is the nurse most likely to suspect in Camille's case?
      a. A psychiatric emergency
      b. A crisis of anticipated life transition
      c. A crisis reflecting psychopathology
    - • d. A crisis resulting from traumatic stress

3. Camille eventually reports that she was nearly raped on Monday night when she took a shortcut on her way from the computer center to her dorm. She is referred to a nurse who is trained as a rape crisis counselor, who schedules appointments three times a

week for 3 weeks. At the first session, Camille announces that she has decided to quit school and return home. What is the most therapeutic response for the counselor to make?

  a. "I'm confident you know what's best for you."
- b. "This is not a good time for you to make such an important decision."
  c. "Your mother and father will be terribly disappointed."
  d. "What will you do if you go home?"

4. In her interventions with Camille, which of the following therapeutic approaches would **best** be implemented by the nurse?

  a. A psychoanalytical approach
  b. A psychodynamic approach
- c. A reality-oriented approach
  d. A family-oriented approach

5. During the final two sessions, Camille and the counselor review the work they have done together. Which of the following statements by Camille would **most** clearly suggest that the goals of crisis intervention have been met?

  a. "Thanks a lot. You've really been helpful. I'll miss working with you."
  b. "My instructor gave me a 3-week extension on my project."
  c. "I'm really glad I didn't go home. It would have been hard to come back."
- d. "I'm wearing the whistle my dad gave me when I go out walking. I've practiced using it, too."

The following questions are related to anger and aggression.

6. Anna is the charge nurse on a psychiatric unit in a large, inner city hospital. She carefully reviews clients' histories when making assignments so that the most experienced staff are assigned to clients who may become violent. Which of the following risk factors does Anna recognize as the **most** reliable indicator for a client becoming violent?

  a. Diagnosis of schizophrenia
- b. Past history of violence
  c. Family history of violence
  d. Tense posture and agitation

7. John, who has a diagnosis of paranoid schizophrenia, is admitted to Anna's unit after attempting to injure his father with a butcher knife. The nurse who writes John's care plan gives him the priority nursing diagnosis: Risk for other-directed violence. Which of the following is the priority goal for John during his hospitalization?

a. The client will not verbalize anger or hit anyone.
b. The client will verbalize anger rather than hit others.
● c. The client will not harm self or others.
d. The client will be restrained if he becomes verbally or physically abusive.

8. Because of the frequency with which they deal with violent clients, the staff on this unit has a violence intervention protocol. Which of the following interventions would be *contraindicated* as part of such a protocol?
a. Administration of psychotropic medication
● b. Soothing the client by stroking an arm or shoulder
c. Application of leather restraints
d. Observation for symptoms of the preassaultive tension state

9. John begins to lose control of his anger, and the nurse decides intervention must occur. John cannot be "talked down," and he refuses medication. The nurse should then:
● a. Call for assistance from the assault team.
b. Ask the ward clerk to put in a call for the physician.
c. Make John go to his room.
d. Tell John if he doesn't calm down, he will be placed in restraints.

10. John is placed in restraints, after which the nurse administers the p.r.n. neuroleptic medication that the client had previously refused. Which of the following statements is true regarding this intervention?
a. The physician must leave a standing order for this intervention to be appropriate.
b. The nurse who intervenes in this manner is setting himself or herself up for a lawsuit, because the client always has a right to refuse medication.
c. The physician must write an order to cover the nurse's actions after the intervention has taken place.
● d. Most states consider this intervention appropriate in emergency situations or if a client would likely harm self or others.

CHAPTER 10. PSYCHOPHARMACOLOGY

CHAPTER FOCUS

The focus of this chapter is to introduce the student to the major drugs used in the psychiatric setting. Those presented include antianxiety agents, antidepressants, mood stabilizers, antipsychotics, antiparkinsonian agents, sedative-hypnotics, and central nervous system stimulants. The role of the nurse in administration of these medications and in client education is emphasized.

LEARNING OBJECTIVES

After reading this chapter, the student will be able to:
1. Discuss historical perspectives related to psychopharmacology.
2. Describe indications, actions, contraindications, precautions, side effects, and nursing implications for the following classifications of drugs:
   a. Antianxiety agents
   b. Antidepressants
   c. Mood stabilizers
   d. Antipsychotics
   e. Antiparkinsonian agents
   f. Sedative-hypnotics
   g. Central nervous system stimulants
3. Apply the steps of the nursing process to the administration of psychotropic medications.

KEY TERMS

hypertensive crisis
priapism
retrograde ejaculation
gynecomastia
amenorrhea
agranulocytosis
extrapyramidal symptoms
akinesia
akathisia
dystonia
oculogyric crisis
tardive dyskinesia
neuroleptic malignant syndrome
serotonin syndrome

CHAPTER OUTLINE/LECTURE NOTES

Copyright © 2002, F. A. Davis Company

I. Historical Perspectives
  A. Neuroleptics were introduced into the United States in the 1950s.
  B. They were intended to be used as an adjunct to individual or group psychotherapy.
II. Applying the Nursing Process in Psychopharmacological Therapy
  A. Antianxiety agents
    1. Background assessment data
      a. Indications: anxiety disorders, anxiety symptoms, acute alcohol withdrawal, skeletal muscle spasms, convulsive disorders, status epilepticus, and preoperative sedation
      b. Examples
      c. Action: depression of the central nervous system
      d. Contraindications/precautions: contraindicated in known hypersensitivity and in combination with other CNS depressants. Caution with elderly and debilitated clients, clients with renal or hepatic dysfunction, clients with a history of drug abuse or addiction, and those who are depressed or suicidal.
      e. Interactions
    2. Diagnoses
      a. Risk for injury
      b. Risk for activity intolerance
      c. Risk for acute confusion
    3. Planning/implementation
      a. Side effects and nursing implications
        (1) Drowsiness, confusion, lethargy
        (2) Tolerance; physical and psychological dependence
        (3) Potentiation of other CNS depressants
        (4) Aggravation of depression
        (5) Orthostatic hypotension
        (6) Paradoxical excitement
        (7) Dry mouth
        (8) Nausea and vomiting
        (9) Blood dyscrasias
        (10) Delayed onset (with buspirone only)
      b. Client/family education
    4. Outcome criteria/evaluation
  B. Antidepressants
    1. Background assessment data
      a. Indications: dysthymic disorder, major depression; depression associated with organic disease, alcoholism, schizophrenia, or mental retardation; depressive phase of bipolar disorder; and depression accompanied by anxiety.
      b. Examples
      c. Action:

        (1) Block the re-uptake of norepinephrine and serotonin by the neurons, thereby increasing their concentrations (tricyclics, tetracyclics, SSRIs)

        (2) Inhibits monoamine oxidase, an enzyme that is known to inactivate norepinephrine, serotonin, and dopamine (MAOIs)

    d. Contraindications/precautions: contraindicated in known hypersensitivity, acute phase of recovery from myocardial infarction, and in angle-closure glaucoma. Caution should be taken in prescribing for elderly, debilitated, or clients with hepatic, cardiac, or renal insufficiency. Caution needed also with psychotic clients, clients with benign prostatic hypertrophy, and those with history of seizures.

    e. Interactions

2. Diagnoses

    a. Risk for suicide

    b. Risk for injury

    c. Social isolation

    d. Constipation

3. Planning/implementation

    a. Side effects and nursing implications

        (1) May occur with all chemical classes:

            (a) Dry mouth

            (b) Sedation

            (c) Nausea

        (2) Most commonly occur with tricyclics or heterocyclics:

            (a) Blurred vision

            (b) Constipation

            (c) Urinary retention

            (d) Orthostatic hypotension

            (e) Reduction of seizure threshold

            (f) Tachycardia; arrhythmias

            (g) Photosensitivity

            (h) Weight gain

        (3) Most commonly occur with SSRIs:

            (a) Insomnia; agitation

            (b) Headache

            (c) Weight loss

            (d) Sexual dysfunction

            (e) **Serotonin syndrome**

        (4) Most commonly occur with MAOIs:

            (a) **Hypertensive crisis**

        (5) Miscellaneous side effects:

            (a) **Priapism** (with trazodone [Desyrel])

    b. Client/family interaction

4. Outcome criteria/evaluation

C. Mood stabilizing agents

1. Background assessment data

a. Indications: prevention and treatment of manic episodes associated with bipolar disorder
b. Examples: lithium carbonate; clonazepam; carbamazepine; valproic acid; verapamil; lamotrigine; gabapentin; topiramate
c. Action: Lithium enhances the re-uptake of norepinephrine and serotonin in the brain, lowering levels in the body and resulting in decreased hyperactivity. The role of the anticonvulsants and verapamil in the treatment of bipolar mania is not fully understood.
d. Interactions
e. Contraindications/precautions

2. Diagnoses
   a. Risk for injury
   b. Risk for violence
   c. Risk for activity intolerance
3. Planning/implementation
   a. Side effects and nursing implications
   b. Lithium toxicity
   c. Client/family education
4. Outcome criteria/evaluation

D. Antipsychotics
1. Background assessment data
   a. Indications: treatment of acute and chronic psychoses. Selected agents are also used as antiemetics, in the treatment of intractable hiccoughs, and for the control of tics and vocal utterances in Tourette's disorder.
   b. Examples
   c. Action: unknown; thought to block postsynaptic dopamine receptors in the basal ganglia, hypothalamus, limbic system, brainstem, and medulla.
   d. Contraindications/precautions: contraindicated with known hypersensitivity, with CNS depression, when blood dyscrasias exist, in clients with Parkinson's disease, or those with liver, renal, or cardiac insufficiency. Caution with elderly, debilitated, or diabetic clients, or those with respiratory insufficiency, prostatic hypertrophy, or intestinal obstruction.
   e. Interactions
2. Diagnoses
   a. Risk for violence
   b. Risk for injury
   c. Risk for activity intolerance
   d. Noncompliance
3. Planning/implementation
   a. Side effects and nursing implications
      (1) Anticholinergic effects
      (2) Nausea; GI upset
      (3) Skin rash
      (4) Sedation

    (5) Orthostatic hypotension

    (6) Photosensitivity

    (7) Hormonal effects

    (8) Reduction of seizure threshold

    (9) **Agranulocytosis**

    (10) Hypersalivation (with Clozapine)

    (11) **Extrapyramidal symptoms** (EPS)

    (12) **Tardive dyskinesia**

    (13) **Neuroleptic malignant syndrome** (NMS)

   b. Client/family education

  4. Outcome criteria/evaluation

E. Antiparkinsonian agents

  1. Background assessment data

   a. Indications: treatment of all forms of parkinsonism and for the relief of drug-induced extrapyramidal reactions

   b. Examples

   c. Action: works to restore the natural balance of acetylcholine and dopamine in the CNS

   d. Contraindications/precautions: contraindicated in known hypersensitivity; angle-closure glaucoma; pyloric, duodenal, or bladder neck obstructions; prostatic hypertrophy; megaesophagus, megacolon, and myasthenia gravis. Caution is advised with hepatic, renal, or cardiac insufficiency; elderly and debilitated clients; those with tendency toward urinary retention; clients exposed to high environmental temperatures; and clients with tachycardia, cardiac arrhythmias, hypertension, or hypotension.

   e. Interactions

  2. Diagnoses

   a. Risk for injury

   b. Hyperthermia

   c. Activity intolerance

   d. Knowledge deficit

  3. Planning/implementation

   a. Side effects

    (1) Anticholinergic effects

    (2) Nausea; GI upset

    (3) Sedation, drowsiness, dizziness

    (4) Exacerbation of psychoses

    (5) Orthostatic hypotension

   b. Client/family education

  4. Outcome criteria/evaluation

F. Sedative-hypnotics

  1. Background assessment data

   a. Indications: short-term management of various anxiety states and to treat insomnia

   b. Examples

    c. Action: depression of the central nervous system

    d. Contraindications/precautions: contraindicated in known hypersensitivity. Caution advised with clients with hepatic dysfunction or severe renal impairment. Caution is also advised with suicidal clients, and clients who have been previously addicted to drugs.

    e. Interactions

  2. Diagnoses

    a. Risk for injury

    b. Sleep pattern disturbance

    c. Risk for activity intolerance

    d. Risk for acute confusion

  3. Planning/Implementation (refer to section on antianxiety medications)

    a. Side effects and nursing implications

    b. Client/family education

  4. Outcome criteria/evaluation

G. Central nervous system (CNS) stimulants

  1. Background assessment data

    a. Indications: in the management of narcolepsy, attention deficit disorder with hyperactivity in children, and as adjunctive therapy to caloric restriction in the treatment of exogenous obesity.

    b. Examples

    c. Action: stimulate the CNS by increasing levels of norepinephrine, dopamine, and serotonin

    d. Contraindications/precautions: contraindicated in individuals with hypersensitivity to sympathomimetic amines; in individuals with advanced arteriosclerosis, symptomatic cardiovascular disease, hypertension, hyperthyroidism, glaucoma, agitated or hyperexcitability states, in clients with a history of drug abuse, during or within 14 days of receiving therapy with MAOIs, in children under 3 years of age, and in pregnancy. Caution during lactation, with psychotic children, in Tourette's disorder, in anorexia or insomnia, in elderly, debilitated, or asthenic clients, and those with a history of suicidal or homicidal tendencies.

    e. Interactions

  2. Diagnoses

    a. Risk for injury

    b. Risk for suicide

    c. Imbalanced nutrition, less than body requirements

    d. Imbalanced nutrition, more than body requirements

    e. Sleep pattern disturbance

  3. Planning/implementation

    a. Side effects and nursing implications

      (1) Overstimulation, restlessness, insomnia

      (2) Palpitations, tachycardia

      (3) Anorexia, weight loss

      (4) Tolerance, physical and psychological dependence

   b. Client/family education
   4. Outcome criteria/evaluation
III. Summary
IV. Review Questions

LEARNING ACTIVITY

PSYCHOTROPIC MEDICATION QUIZ

Please fill in the blanks and answer the questions in the space provided:

1. What is the mechanism of action by which antidepressant medications achieve the desired effect (regardless of the different physiological processes by which this action is accomplished)?

2. For what must the nurse be on the alert with the client who is receiving antidepressant medication?

3. As the nurse, when would you expect the client to begin showing signs of symptomatic relief after the initiation of antidepressant therapy?

4. Name an example of a tricyclic antidepressant._____
  Name an example of an MAOI._____
  Name an example of an SSRI._____

5. Describe some common side effects of and nursing implications for tricyclic antidepressants.

6. _____ is the most potentially life-threatening adverse effect of MAO inhibitors. Symptoms for which the nurse and client must be on the alert include: _____ _____. What must be done to prevent these symptoms from occurring? (Your answer must include some examples.)

7. Lithium carbonate is the drug of choice for _____. Many times when these individuals are started on lithium therapy, the physician also orders an antipsychotic medication. Why might he or she do so?

8. There is a narrow margin between the therapeutic and toxic serum levels of lithium carbonate. What is the therapeutic range, and list the initial signs and symptoms of lithium toxicity.

9. Describe some nursing implications for the client on lithium therapy.

10. What is the mechanism of action for antianxiety medications?

11. What is the most commonly used group of antianxiety drugs? Give two examples.

12. What are the most common side effects of antianxiety drugs?

13. What must the client on long-term antianxiety therapy be instructed to do in order to prevent a potentially life-threatening situation?

14. What is the mechanism of action that produces the desired effect with antipsychotic medications (regardless of the physiological process by which this action is accomplished)?

15. Phenothiazines are the most commonly used antipsychotic group. Give two examples of phenothiazines.

16. Describe potential adverse hormonal effects associated with antipsychotic therapy.

17. Agranulocytosis is a potentially very serious side effect of antipsychotic therapy. The nurse and client should be on the alert for symptoms of _____, _____, and _____.

18. Neuroleptic malignant syndrome (NMS) is a rare, but potentially fatal, side effect of antipsychotic drugs. List symptoms for which the nurse must be on the alert when assessing for NMS.

19. Describe the symptoms of extrapyramidal side effects associated with antipsychotic therapy.

20. What is the classification of medication that is commonly prescribed for drug-induced extrapyramidal reactions? Give two examples of these medications.

21. Describe a life-threatening situation that could occur in the client who abruptly withdraws from long-term use of CNS stimulants.

TEST QUESTIONS

1. Carol has made an appointment to see her primary care provider because of increased anxiety. She sees a nurse practitioner who does a physical examination and takes a detailed history. The psychiatrist diagnoses Carol with anxiety disorder. Which of the following medications is prescribed for anxiety?
    a. chlorpromazine (Thorazine)
    b. amitriptyline (Elavil)
 • c. diazepam (Valium)
    d. methylphenidate (Ritalin)

2. Which of the following data would suggest that caution is necessary in prescribing the medication of choice to Carol?
 • a. The client has a history of alcohol dependence.
    b. The client has a history of diabetes mellitus.
    c. The client has a history of schizophrenia.
    d. The client has a history of hypertension.

3. Peter has been diagnosed with major depression. His psychiatrist prescribes imipramine (Tofranil). What information is specifically related to *this* class of antidepressants and should be included in client/family education?
    a. The medication may cause dry mouth.
    b. The medication may cause constipation.
    c. The medication should not be discontinued abruptly.

- d. The medication may cause photosensitivity.

4. When Peter did not achieve relief from his depression, his psychiatrist decided to try Parnate, an MAOI. When teaching Peter about the effects of tyramine, which of the following foods and/or medications will the nurse caution Peter not to consume?
- a. Pepperoni pizza and red wine
    b. Bagels with cream cheese and tea
    c. Apple pie and coffee
    d. Potato chips and diet coke

5. Alex, a 24-year-old graduate student, is taken to the emergency department by one of his classmates because of increased suspiciousness and auditory hallucinations. He keeps asking others what they are whispering about him. The nurse who takes his history discovers that he has a history of depression, and has been taking desipramine (Norpramine) for 3 years. He is in good physical health, but has allergies to penicillin, compazine, and bee stings. Although a definitive diagnosis is not made, it is clear that Alex is experiencing a psychotic episode. Using the assessment data gathered upon admission, which of the following antipsychotic medications would be contraindicated for Alex?
    a. Haloperidol (Haldol)
    b. Clozapine (Clozaril)
    c. Risperidone (Risperdal)
- d. Thioridazine (Mellaril)

6. Which of the following is the rationale for the correct answer in the previous question?
- a. Cross-sensitivity is common among the phenothiazines.
    b. The drug is new and not adequately tested.
    c. The drug is old and more effective ones have been developed.
    d. It is one of the phenothiazines that is least effective for the treatment of psychosis.

7. The physician prescribes a medication for Alex described as "p.r.n. for EPS." When should the nurse give this medication?
    a. When Alex's white cell count falls below 3000 mm^3
- b. When Alex exhibits tremors and shuffling gait
    c. When Alex complains of dry mouth
    d. When Alex experiences a seizure

8. Which of the following medications would the physician have prescribed for the EPS described in the previous question?
    a. Diazepam (Valium)
    b. Amitriptyline (Elavil)
  • c. Benztropine (Cogentin)
    d. Methylphenidate (Ritalin)

9. Nancy takes a maintenance dosage of lithium carbonate for a history of bipolar disorder. She has come to the community health clinic stating that she "has had the flu for over a week." She describes her symptoms as coughing, runny nose, chest congestion, fever, and GI upset. Her temperature is 100.9° F. She is complaining of blurred vision and "ringing in my ears." What might the nurse suspect in Nancy's case?
    a. She has consumed some foods high in tyramine.
    b. She has stopped taking her lithium carbonate.
    c. She has probably developed a tolerance to the lithium.
  • d. She may have become toxic on the lithium carbonate.

10. Joey, age 8, takes methylphenidate (Ritalin) for ADHD. His mother complains to the nurse that Joey has a very poor appetite, and she struggles to help him gain weight. Which of the following would be appropriate for the nurse to advise Joey's mother?
  • a. Administer Joey's medication immediately after meals.
    b. Administer Joey's medication at bedtime.
    c. Skip a dose of the medication when Joey doesn't eat anything.
    d. Assure Joey's mother that Joey will eat when he is hungry.

CHAPTER 11. COMPLEMENTARY THERAPIES

CHAPTER FOCUS

The focus of this chapter is to introduce the student to various alternatives to allopathic medicine. The historical background and techniques of each are presented.

LEARNING OBJECTIVES

After reading this chapter, the student will be able to:
1. Describe the philosophies behind various complementary therapies, including herbal medicine, acupressure and acupuncture, diet and nutrition, chiropractic medicine, therapeutic touch and massage, yoga, and pet therapy.
2. Discuss the historical background of various complementary therapies.
3. Describe the techniques used in various complementary therapies.

KEY TERMS

allopathic medicine
alternative medicine
complementary medicine
acupressure
acupuncture
acupoints
chiropractic
subluxation
chi
meridians
yoga

CHAPTER OUTLINE/LECTURE NOTES
I. Introduction
    A. The connection between mind and body is well recognized.
    B. Traditional medicine practiced in the United States today is based on scientific methodology and is known as **allopathic medicine**.
    C. Practices that differ from the usual traditional practices are known as **alternative medicine**.
    D. The Office of Alternative Medicine was established by the National Institutes of Health in 1991 to study nontraditional therapies and to evaluate their usefulness and their effectiveness.
    E. Increasing numbers of third-party payers are bowing to public pressure and including alternative therapies in their coverage.
    F. Some clinicians view these therapies not as alternatives, but as complementary therapies, in partnership with traditional medicine.

G. **Complementary medicine** is viewed as holistic health care, which deals not only with the physical perspective, but also the emotional and spiritual components of the individual.

H. Most complementary therapies are not founded in scientific principle, but they have been shown to be effective in the treatment of certain disorders, and, therefore, merit further examination as a viable component of holistic health care.

I. A table of commonalities and contrasts between complementary medicine and conventional health care is included.

II. Types of Complementary Therapies

A. Herbal medicine
1. Virtually every culture in the world has relied on herbs and plants to treat illness.
2. Twenty-five percent of all prescription drugs in the United States today are derived from plants.
3. The Food and Drug Administration (FDA) classifies herbal remedies as dietary supplements or food additives. Therefore their labels cannot indicate medicinal uses, and they are not subjected to FDA approval.
4. The Commission E of the German Federal Health Agency has been researching and regulating the safety and efficacy of herbs and plant medicines in Germany. Recently, all 380 German Commission E monographs of herbal medicines have been translated into English.
5. Just because a substance is called "natural" does not mean that it is necessarily completely safe. All herbal medicines must be approached with caution.
6. The following cautions are offered:
   a. Be careful of sources.
   b. Choose the most reliable forms.
   c. More is not better.
   d. Monitor your reactions.
   e. Take no risks by self-medicating with herbal remedies.
7. Examples of herbal medicines, their uses, action, and safety profile are included.

B. **Acupressure** and **acupuncture**
1. Acupressure and acupuncture are healing techniques based on the ancient philosophies of traditional Chinese medicine dating back to 3000 B.C.
2. The main concept is that healing energy (**chi**) flows through the body along specific pathways called **meridians**. The meridians connect a series of **acupoints** to which the clinician applies pressure.
3. Pressure to these acupoints is thought to dissolve any obstructions in the flow of healing energy (chi), and to restore the body to a healthier functioning.
4. In acupuncture, hair-thin, sterile, disposable, stainless-steel needles are inserted into acupoints to dissolve the obstructions along the meridians.
5. The Western medical philosophy regarding acupressure and acupuncture is that they stimulate the body's own painkilling chemicals, the morphine-line substances known as endorphins.

6. The treatment has been found to be effective in the treatment of asthma, headaches, dysmenorrhea, cervical pain, insomnia, anxiety, depression, substance abuse, stroke rehabilitation, nausea of pregnancy, postoperative and chemotherapy-induced nausea and vomiting, tennis elbow, fibromyalgia, low back pain, and carpal tunnel syndrome.

C. Diet and nutrition
  1. Many diseases today are linked to poor nutritional habits.
  2. The U.S. Departments of Agriculture and Health and Human Services have collaborated on a set of guidelines to help individuals understand what types of foods to eat in order to promote health and prevent disease. They include:
    a. Eat a variety of foods. Most of the daily servings of food should be selected from the food groups that comprise the largest area and are closest to the base of the food pyramid.
    b. Balance the food you eat with physical activity to maintain or improve your weight. Thirty minutes or more of moderate physical activity (such as walking) 3 to 5 days a week can help to increase calorie expenditure and assist in maintaining a healthy weight.
    c. Choose a diet with plenty of grain products, vegetables, and fruits. Consumption of these foods is associated with a substantially lower risk for many chronic diseases, including certain types of cancer.
    d. Choose a diet low in fat, saturated fat, and cholesterol. Heart disease and some types of cancer (for example, breast and colon) have been linked to high-fat diets. Choose foods with mono- and polyunsaturated fat sources, and keep daily cholesterol intake below 300 mg. Fats should comprise no more than 30 percent of the total daily calorie intake.
    e. Choose a diet moderate in sugars. Sugars should be used in moderation by most healthy people and sparingly by people with low calorie needs. Problems correlated with eating sugar include tooth decay and the risk for heart disease in women 35 and older.
    f. Choose a diet moderate in salt and sodium. Some studies indicate that a high intake of salt is associated with high blood pressure.
    g. If you drink alcoholic beverages, do so in moderation. High levels of alcohol intake raise the risk for high blood pressure, stroke, heart disease, certain cancers, accidents, violence, suicides, birth defects, cirrhosis of the liver, inflammation of the pancreas, damage to the brain, and overall mortality.
  3. Essential vitamins and minerals
    a. Examples
    b. Functions
    c. RDA requirements
    d. Food sources

D. **Chiropractic** medicine
  1. Chiropractic medicine is probably the most widely used form of alternative healing in the United States. It was developed in the late 1800s.

2. Theory behind this type of healing is that energy flows from the brain to all parts of the body through the spinal cord and spinal nerves. When vertebrae of the spinal column become displaced, they may press on a nerve and interfere with the normal nerve transmission.
3. Displacements of vertebrae are called "**subluxations**." To restore normal function, the vertebrae are manipulated back into their normal positions.
4. The manipulations are called *adjustments*.
5. Adjustments are made by hand or facilitated by the use of special treatment tables.
6. Muscle relaxation may be achieved with massage, the application of heat or cold, and through the use of ultrasound treatments.
7. The most common type of ailment for which individuals seek chiropractic treatment is back pain. Others include headaches, sciatica, shoulder pain, tennis and golfer's elbow, leg and foot pain, hand and wrist pain, allergies, asthma, stomach disorders, and menstrual problems.
8. Chiropractors are licensed to practice in all 50 states.

E. Therapeutic touch and massage
1. The technique of therapeutic touch was developed in the 1970s by Dolores Krieger, a nurse associated with the New York University School of Nursing.
2. This therapy is based on the philosophy that the human body projects a field of energy around it, which when blocked, produces pain or illness.
3. Therapeutic touch is used to correct the blockages and relieve the discomfort.
4. Because therapeutic touch is based on the premise that the energy field extends beyond the surface of the body, the practitioner need not actually touch the client's skin.
5. Slow, rhythmic hand motions are swept over the entire body while the hands remain 2 to 4 inches from the skin. Heat should be felt where the energy is blocked.
6. The therapist "massages" the energy field in that area, smoothing it out, and thus correcting the obstruction.
7. Therapeutic touch is thought to reduce pain and anxiety and to promote relaxation and health maintenance. It has been useful in the treatment of chronic health conditions.

F. Massage
1. Massage is the technique of manipulating the muscles and soft tissues of the body.
2. Chinese physicians prescribed massage for the treatment of disease more than 5000 years ago.
3. The Eastern style of massage focuses on balancing the body's vital energy (chi) as it flows through pathways called meridians.
4. The Western style of massage affects muscles, connective tissues, such as tendons and ligaments, and the cardiovascular system.
5. A variety of gliding and kneading strokes, along with deep circular movements and vibrations, are used to relax the muscles, improve circulation, and increase mobility.

6. Massage is helpful in reducing anxiety, and in relieving chronic back and neck pain, arthritis, sciatica, migraine headaches, muscle spasms, insomnia, pain of labor and delivery, stress-related disorders, and whiplash.
7. Massage is contraindicated in high blood pressure, acute infection, osteoporosis, phlebitis, skin conditions, varicose veins, or over the site of a recent injury, bruises, or burns.

G. **Yoga**
1. Yoga is thought to have been developed in India some 5000 years ago.
2. The ultimate goal of yoga is to unite the human soul with the universal spirit.
3. Yoga is helpful in relieving stress and in improving overall physical and psychological wellness.
4. Yoga breathing is a deep, diaphramatic breathing that increases oxygen to brain and body tissues, thereby easing stress and fatigue, and boosting energy.
5. Another component of yoga is meditation, used to achieve a profound feeling of relaxation.
6. Western yoga uses body postures, along with meditation and breathing exercises, to achieve a balanced, disciplined workout that releases muscle tension, tones the internal organs, and energizes the mind, body, and spirit, so that natural healing can occur.

H. Pet therapy
1. Evidence has shown that animals can directly influence a person's mental and physical well-being.
2. Pets have been shown to:
   a. Reduce the death rate from recurrence of heart attack.
   b. Lower blood pressure, which can occur simply by petting a dog or cat.
   c. Enhance mood and improve social interaction among nursing home clients.
3. Some researchers believe that animals actually may retard the aging process among those who live alone.

III. Summary
IV. Review Questions

LEARNING ACTIVITY

Fill in the food pyramid with the appropriate food groups for each level and the number of servings suggested for each group.

Food Group:
No. of Servings:

Food Group: Food Group:
No. of Servings: No. of Servings:

Food Group: Food Group:
No.of Servings: No. of Servings:

Food Group:
No. of Servings:

TEST QUESTIONS

1. Carol went to the community mental health clinic because she was feeling depressed. She told the therapist that she had broken up with her boyfriend 6 weeks ago, and she has been feeling depressed since that time. She wants to feel better, but she doesn't want to take medication. She told the therapist she would be willing to take an herbal medication if there was something that might help her feel better. The therapist may suggest which of the following for Carol?
   a. Chamomile
   b. Echinacea
   - c. St. John's wort
   d. Feverfew

2. Carol decided to see a chiropractor for a recurring pain in her lower back. The chiropractor took x-rays and told Carol he saw some displacement of vertebrae in her spine. In chiropractic medicine, these displacements are called:
   a. Maladjustments
   b. Manipulations
   c. Meridians
   - d. Subluxations

3. The therapist suggested that Carol see a physician for a complete physical examination. Part of the examination included a health risk assessment. Carol's medical history revealed that her father had died of colon cancer and her mother has had surgery for breast cancer, both of which may have a nutritional link. The nurse does health teaching about diet with Carol. In terms of her risk factors, which of the following food groups should Carol modify her intake of?
   a. Fruit group
   - b. Fats, oils and sweets group
   c. Milk, yogurt and cheese group
   d. Bread, cereal, rice and pasta group

4. Which of the following herbal remedies is thought to improve memory and blood circulation?
   - a. Ginkgo
   b. Ginseng
   c. Kava-Kava
   d. St. John's Wort

5. The technique of yoga uses which of the following?
   a. Deep breathing
   b. Meditation
   c. Balanced body postures
 • d. All of the above

6. Nancy is seeing the nurse practitioner and complains of having trouble sleeping. Which of the following herbal remedies might the nurse prescribe for Nancy?
   a. Ginkgo
   b. Ginseng
 • c. Valerian
   d. Feverfew

7. Recent research has shown that sugar may be a risk factor for women 35 and older in the development of:
   a. Diabetes.
 • b. Heart disease.
   c. Breast cancer.
   d. Osteoporosis.

8. Massage is contraindicated in which of the following conditions?
   a. Arthritis
   b. Migraine headaches
   c. Muscle spasms
 • d. Phlebitis

9. Research indicates that which of the following alternative strategies has been shown to lower blood pressure:
 • a. Petting a dog or cat.
   b. Chiropractic adjustments.
   c. High doses of magnesium.
   d. Drinking chamomile tea.

10. Which of the following herbal remedies is thought to stimulate the immune system and ease the symptoms of colds and flu?
    a. Ginseng
    b. Kava-Kava
 • c. Echinacea

d. Valerian

CHAPTER 12. DELIRIUM, DEMENTIA, AND AMNESTIC DISORDERS

CHAPTER FOCUS

The focus of this chapter is on etiological implications, symptomatology, and nursing interventions for the care of clients with delirium, dementia, and amnestic disorders. These disorders were identified in previous editions of the *Diagnostic and Statistical Manual of Mental Disorders (DSM)* as organic mental syndromes and disorders.

LEARNING OBJECTIVES

After reading this chapter, the student will be able to:
1. Define and differentiate among *delirium, dementia,* and *amnestic disorder.*
2. Discuss etiological implications of delirium, dementia, and amnestic disorders.
3. Describe clinical symptoms and use the information to assess clients with delirium, dementia, and amnestic disorders.
4. Identify nursing diagnoses common to clients with delirium, dementia, and amnestic disorders, and select appropriate nursing interventions for each.
5. Identify topics for client and family teaching relevant to these disorders.
6. Discuss criteria for evaluating nursing care of clients with delirium, dementia, and amnestic disorders.
7. Describe various treatment modalities relevant to care of clients with delirium, dementia, and amnestic disorders.

KEY TERMS

amnestic disorders
aphasia
apraxia
ataxia
confabulation
delirium
dementia
pseudodementia
primary dementia
secondary dementia

CHAPTER OUTLINE/LECTURE NOTES

I. Introduction
    A. This chapter discusses disorders in which a clinically significant deficit in cognition or memory exists, representing a significant change from a previous level of functioning.

B. The number of individuals with these disorders is growing because more people now survive into the high-risk period for **dementia** of middle age and beyond.

II. **Delirium**

A. Characterized by a disturbance of consciousness and change in cognition that develop rapidly over a short period.

B. Symptoms include:
1. Difficulty sustaining and shifting attention.
2. Extreme distractibility.
3. Disorganized thinking.
4. Speech that is rambling, irrelevant, pressured, and incoherent.
5. Impaired reasoning ability and goal-directed behavior.
6. Disorientation to time and place.
7. Impairment of recent memory.
8. Misperceptions of the environment, including illusions and hallucinations.
9. Disturbance in level of consciousness, with interruption of the sleep-wake cycle.
10. Psychomotor activity that fluctuates between agitation and restlessness and a vegetative state.
11. Emotional instability.
12. Autonomic manifestations, such as tachycardia, sweating, flushed face, dilated pupils, and elevated blood pressure.

C. Delirium usually begins abruptly, for instance, following a head injury or seizure. It can have a slower onset if the underlying etiology is systemic illness or metabolic imbalance.

D. Duration is usually brief (for example, 1 week; rarely more than 1 month) and subsides completely on recovery from the underlying determinant.

E. Etiological implications
1. Delirium due to a general medical condition, such as systemic infections, metabolic disorders (for example, hypoxia, hypercarbia, and hypoglycemia), fluid or electrolyte imbalances, hepatic or renal disease, thiamine deficiency, postoperative states, hypertensive encephalopathy, postictal states, and sequelae of head trauma.
2. Substance-induced delirium. Symptoms are attributed to side effects of certain medications or exposure to a toxin. Medications that may produce these symptoms include anesthetics, analgesics, antiasthmatic agents, anticonvulsants, antihistamines, antihypertensive and cardiovascular medications, antimicrobials, antiparkinsonian agents, neuroleptics, corticosteroids, gastrointestinal medications, histamine H_2-receptor antagonists (for example, cimetidine), immunosuppressive agents, lithium, muscle relaxants, and psychotropic medications with anticholinergic side effects. Toxins reported to cause delirium include organophosphates (anticholinesterase), insecticides, carbon monoxide, and volatile substances such as fuel or organic solvents.

3. Substance-intoxication delirium. Symptoms may occur following ingestion of high doses of cannabis, cocaine, hallucinogens, alcohol, anxiolytics, or narcotics.
4. Substance-withdrawal delirium. Withdrawal delirium symptoms develop after reduction or termination of sustained, usually high-dose use of certain substances such as alcohol, sedatives, hypnotics, or anxiolytics.
5. Delirium due to multiple etiologies. The delirium symptoms may be related to more than one general medical condition or to the combined effects of a general medical condition and substance use.

III. Dementia
 A. Defined as a syndrome of acquired, persistent intellectual impairment with compromised function in multiple spheres of mental activity, such as memory, language, visuospatial skills, emotion or personality, and cognition.
 B. Dementias can be classified as either primary or secondary.
  1. **Primary dementia**—the dementia itself is the major sign of some organic brain disease, such as Alzheimer's disease.
  2. **Secondary dementia**—the dementia is caused by, or related to, another disease or condition, such as HIV disease or a cerebral trauma.
 C. Symptoms include:
  1. Impairment in abstract thinking, judgment, and impulse control.
  2. Disregard for the conventional rules of social conduct.
  3. Neglect of personal appearance and hygiene.
  4. Effects on language (not always).
  5. Changes in personality (common, but not always).
 D. Truly reversible dementia occurs in only 2 to 3 percent of cases and is determined by the underlying pathology and timely application of effective treatment.
 E. As the disease progresses, symptoms may include:
  1. **Aphasia** (absence of speech).
  2. **Apraxia** (inability to carry out motor activities despite intact motor functioning).
  3. Irritability and moodiness, with sudden outbursts over trivial issues.
  4. Inability to care for personal needs independently.
  5. Wandering away from the home.
  6. Incontinence.
 F. Dementia of the Alzheimer's type (DAT) accounts for about 50 to 60 percent of all cases of dementia. DAT progresses according to stages:
  1. Stage 1: No apparent symptoms.
  2. Stage 2: Forgetfulness. Experiences loss of short-term memory. Anxiety and depression common.
  3. Stage 3: Early confusion. Has difficulty concentrating. Individual may become lost while driving.
  4. Stage 4: Late confusion. Forgets important dates. Unable to perform tasks or understand current events. May use **confabulation**.

5. Stage 5: Early dementia. Unable to perform activities of daily living independently. May forget names of close relatives. Requires assistance to manage on an ongoing basis.

6. Stage 6. Middle dementia. May be unable to recall recent major life events, or even name of spouse. Disoriented to time and place. Incontinence, agitation, and sleeping may be a problem. Wandering is common. Institutional care is usually required at this time.

7. Late dementia. Unable to recognize family. Commonly bedfast and aphasic.

G. Etiological implications:
   1. Dementia of the Alzheimer's type.
      a. Onset is slow and insidious and the course of the disorder is generally progressive and deteriorating.
      b. Definitive diagnosis requires biopsy or autopsy examination of brain tissue.
      c. Etiologies may include:
         (1) Acetylcholine alterations.
         (2) Accumulation of aluminum.
         (3) Alterations in the immune system.
         (4) Head trauma.
         (5) Genetic factors.
   2. Vascular dementia.
      a. Dementia is due to significant cerebrovascular disease (significant number of small strokes).
      b. There is a more abrupt onset than is seen in Alzheimer's disease, and the course is more variable.
      c. Etiologies may include:
         (1) Arterial hypertension.
         (2) Cerebral emboli.
         (3) Cerebral thrombosis.
   3. Dementia due to HIV disease
      a. Dementia is due to brain infections by opportunistic organisms or by the HIV-1 virus directly.
      b. Symptoms may range from barely perceptible changes to acute delirium to profound dementia.
   4. Dementia due to head trauma
      a. Posttrauma symptoms include headache, irritability, dizziness, diminished concentration, and hypersensitivity to certain stimuli.
      b. Intellectual functioning and memory may also be impaired.
   5. Dementia due to Parkinson's disease
      a. This dementia is caused by a loss of nerve cells located in the substantia nigra, and a decrease in dopamine activity.
      b. Cerebral changes in dementia of Parkinson's sometimes resemble those of Alzheimer's disease.
   6. Dementia due to Huntington's disease

a. Damage from this disease occurs in the areas of the basal ganglia and the cerebral cortex.

b. A profound state of dementia and **ataxia** occurs within 5 to 10 years of onset.

7. Dementia due to Pick's disease

   a. Pathology results from atrophy in the frontal and temporal lobes of the brain.

   b. Clinical picture is very similar to that of Alzheimer's disease.

8. Dementia due to Creutzfeldt-Jacob disease

   a. Onset of symptoms occurs between ages 40 and 60, and the course is extremely rapid with progressive deterioration and death within 1 year.

   b. Etiology is thought to be a transmissible agent known as a "slow virus." Five to 15 percent of cases have a genetic component.

9. Dementia due to other general medical conditions

   a. Other medical conditions that can cause dementia include:

      (1) Endocrine conditions

      (2) Pulmonary disease

      (3) Hepatic or renal failure

      (4) Cardiopulmonary insufficiency

      (5) Fluid and electrolyte imbalances

      (6) Nutritional deficiencies

      (7) Frontal or temporal lobe lesions

      (8) Central nervous system or systemic infections

      (9) Uncontrolled epilepsy

      (10) Other neurological conditions, such as multiple sclerosis

10. Substance-induced persisting dementia

    a. Dementia is related to the persisting effects of use of substances such as:

       (1) Alcohol

       (2) Inhalants

       (3) Sedatives, hypnotics, and anxiolytics

       (4) Medications, such as anticonvulsants and intrathecal methotrexate

       (5) Toxins, such as lead, mercury, carbon monoxide, organophosphate insecticides, and industrial solvents

11. Dementia due to multiple etiologies

    a. This diagnosis is used when the symptoms of dementia are attributed to more than one etiology.

IV. **Amnestic Disorders**

A. Amnestic disorders are characterized by an inability to learn new information (short-term memory deficit) despite normal attention, and an inability to recall previously learned information (long-term memory deficit).

B. Other symptoms include:

   1. Disorientation to place and time (rarely to self).

   2. Confabulation, the creation of imaginary events to fill in memory gaps.

   3. Denial that a problem exists, or acknowledgment that a problem exists, but with a lack of concern.

4. Apathy, lack of initiative, and emotional blandness.
C. Onset may be acute or insidious, depending on the underlying pathological process.
D. Duration and course may be quite variable and are also correlated with extent and severity of the cause.
E. Etiological implications
  1. Amnestic disorder due to a general medical condition. Medical conditions that may be associated with amnestic disorder include:
    a. Head trauma.
    b. Cerebrovascular disease.
    c. Cerebral neoplastic disease.
    d. Cerebral anoxia.
    e. Herpes simplex encephalitis.
    f. Poorly controlled insulin-dependent diabetes.
    g. Surgical intervention to the brain.
  2. Transient amnestic syndromes can occur from:
    a. Epileptic seizures.
    b. Electroconvulsive therapy.
    c. Severe migraine headache.
    d. Drug overdose.
  3. Substance-induced persisting amnestic disorder. The amnestic symptoms are related to the persisting effects of the use of the following substances:
    a. Alcohol.
    b. Sedatives, hypnotics, and anxiolytics.
    c. Medications, such as anticonvulsants and intrathecal methotrexate.
    d. Toxins, such as lead, mercury, carbon monoxide, organophosphate insecticides, and industrial solvents.
V. Application of the Nursing Process
  A. The client history
    1. The following areas of concern should be addressed:
      a. Type, frequency, and severity of mood swings.
      b. Personality and behavioral changes.
      c. Catastrophic emotional reactions.
      d. Cognitive changes.
      e. Language difficulties.
      f. Orientation to person, place, time, and situation.
      g. Appropriateness of social behavior.
      h. Current and past use of medications.
      i. Current and past use of drugs and alcohol.
      j. Possible exposure to toxins.
      k. Client/family history of specific illnesses.
  B. Physical assessment
    1. Assessment for diseases of various organ systems that can induce confusion, loss of memory, and behavioral changes

2. Neurological examination to assess mental status, alertness, muscle strength, reflexes, sensory perception, language skills, and coordination
3. Psychological tests to differentiate between dementia and **pseudodementia** (depression)

C. Diagnostic laboratory evaluations
 1. Possible laboratory evaluations include blood and urine evaluations to test for:
   a. Various infections.
   b. Hepatic and renal dysfunction.
   c. Diabetes or hypoglycemia.
   d. Electrolyte imbalances.
   e. Metabolic and endocrine disorders.
   f. Nutritional deficiencies.
   g. Presence of toxic substances, including alcohol and drugs.
 2. Other diagnostic evaluations may include:
   a. Electroencephalogram (EEG).
   b. Computerized tomography (CT) scan.
   c. Positron emission tomography (PET).
   d. Magnetic resonance imaging (MRI).
   e. Lumbar puncture to examine cerebrospinal fluid.

B. Diagnosis/outcome identification
 1. Common nursing diagnoses for the client with cognitive dysfunction include:
   a. Risk for trauma.
   b. Risk for suicide.
   c. Risk for other-directed violence.
   d. Altered thought processes.
   e. Self-esteem disturbance.
   f. Self-care deficit.

C. Planning/implementation
D. Client/family education
E. Evaluation

VI. Medical Treatment Modalities
 A. Delirium
  1. Determination and correction of the underlying causes
  2. Staff should remain with client at all times to monitor behavior and provide reorientation and assurance.
  3. Room with low level of stimuli.
  4. Low-dose neuroleptics (for example, haloperidol) to relieve agitation and aggression.
 B. Dementia
  1. Primary consideration is given to etiology, with focus on identification and resolution of potentially reversible processes.
  2. A number of pharmaceutical agents have been tried with varying degrees of success in the treatment of dementia. They include:
   a. For cognitive impairment:
    (1) Physostigmine (Antilirium)

        (2) Cyclandelate (Cyclan)

        (3) Ergoloid mesylate (Hydergine)

        (4) Tacrine (Cognex)

        (5) Donepezil (Aricept)

        (6) Rivastigmine (Exelon)

    b. For agitation, aggression, hallucinations, thought disturbances, and wandering:

        (1) Thiothixene (Navane)

        (2) Chlorpromazine (Thorazine)

        (3) Thioridazine (Mellaril)

        (4) Haloperidol (Haldol)

    c. For depression:

        (1) Amitriptyline (Elavil)

        (2) Desipramine (Norpramine)

        (3) Doxepin (Adapin)

        (4) Imipramine (Tofranil)

        (5) Trazodone (Desyrel)

        (6) Bupropion (Wellbutrin)

        (7) Fluoxetine (Prozac)

        (8) Paroxitine (Paxil)

        (9) Sertraline (Zoloft)

    d. For anxiety (these medications should not be used routinely or for prolonged periods):

        (1) Diazepam (Valium)

        (2) Chlordiazepoxide (Librium)

        (3) Alprazolam (Xanax)

        (4) Lorazepam (Ativan)

        (5) Oxazepam (Serax)

    e. For sleep disturbances (for short-term therapy only):

        (1) Flurazepam (Dalmane)

        (2) Temazepam (Restoril)

        (3) Triazolam (Halcion)

VII. Summary

VIII. Critical Thinking Exercise

IX. Review Questions

ANSWERS TO CRITICAL THINKING EXERCISE

1. Anxiety, confusion, disorientation, physically abusive, suspiciousness

2. Risk for trauma related to confusion and disorientation

3. Outcomes would be based on short-term goals. Because the disease is progressive, it would be unrealistic to expect resolution, so a series of step-objectives would be used. For example:

Goal: Joe will not harm himself in his confused state.
Outcome criteria:

1. Joe is allowed to wander in a safe, enclosed area.
2. Joe is able to find his room with the aid of a large sign on the door that identifies it by name.

Goal: Joe will be able to perform self-care needs with assistance.
Outcome criteria:

1. Joe washes his face with supplies provided by the nurse.
2. Joe dresses himself with step-instructions from the nurse.
3. Joe straightens up his room with direction from the nurse.

CASE STUDY FOR USE WITH STUDENT LEARNING

Case Study: <u>Dementia of the Alzheimer's Type</u>

Gary received a call at work recently from the police in the small town where he lived and worked. They told him that they had picked up his father, George, age 69, whom they found wandering about 10 blocks from his home. George told the police he did not remember where he lived. George, a former banker in the small town, was well known to most of the citizens. Gary retrieved his father from the police station and took him home. He and his mother made an appointment to have George evaluated. George's wife reported to the physician that George had grown progressively more forgetful over the last few years; however, they had just been laughing it off as "old age." A physical examination and MRI were conducted, resulting with the physician's diagnosis of dementia of the Alzheimer's type. A home health nurse was assigned as case manager for George and his wife to manage the progression of his illness. Design a plan of care in the management of George's illness by the nursing case manager.

LEARNING ACTIVITY

DELIRIUM, DEMENTIA, AND AMNESTIC DISORDERS

Check whether the behaviors described on the left are characteristic of delirium, dementia, or amnestic disorder. (Each may apply to more than one condition.)

	Delirium	Dementia	Amnestic Disorder
1. Duration of the disorder is commonly brief.	___	___	___
2. Client uses confabulation to hide cognitive deficits.	___	___	___
3. Symptoms may be confused with depression.	___	___	___
4. Can be caused by a series of small strokes.	___	___	___
5. Is commonly reversible.	___	___	___

6. Denial that a problem exists is common. ___ ___ ___

7. Level of consciousness is affected. ___ ___ ___

8. Reversibility occurs in only 2 to 3 percent of cases. ___ ___ ___

9. Severe migraine headache can cause transient symptoms. ___ ___ ___

10. Personality change is common. ___ ___ ___

11. Illusions and hallucinations are common symptoms. ___ ___ ___

12. Symptoms can occur as a result of cocaine intoxication. ___ ___ ___

13. Symptoms can occur as a result of alcohol withdrawal. ___ ___ ___

14. High concentrations of aluminum in the brain have been implicated in the etiology of this disorder. ___ ___ ___

15. Transient symptoms of this disorder can occur following electroconvulsive therapy. ___ ___ ___

TEST QUESTIONS

Gloria visits her Aunt Naomi about twice a year. Naomi is 74 years old and lives in a city about 300 miles away from Gloria. During her most recent visit, Gloria notices that her aunt has become quite forgetful. Two days worth of mail are still in the mailbox, and Naomi has forgotten to have her prescription for her antihypertensive medication refilled. There is very little food in the house, and Naomi is unable to tell Gloria when or what she last ate. Gloria calls Naomi's physician, who has Naomi hospitalized for evaluation.

1. The physician diagnoses Naomi with dementia. From the information given, which of the following types of dementia does Naomi most likely have?
    a. Dementia of the Alzheimer's type
  • b. Vascular dementia
    c. Dementia due to head trauma
    d. Dementia due to Parkinson's disease

2. Which of the following statements is true about this type of dementia?
    a. It is reversible.
    b. It is characterized by plaques and tangles in the brain.
    c. It exhibits a gradual, progressive deterioration.

- d. It exhibits a fluctuating pattern of deterioration.

3. The physician orders cyclandelate (Cyclan) for Naomi. The rationale for this order is:
    - a. To enhance circulation to the brain.
    - b. To elevate levels of acetylcholine in the brain.
    - c. To control aggressive behavior.
    - d. To prevent depression.

4. Which of the following nursing diagnoses would be a *priority* for the nurse caring for Naomi?
    - a. Altered thought processes
    - b. Self-care deficit
    - c. Risk for trauma
    - d. Risk for violence toward others

5. The physician tells Gloria that it is not safe for Naomi to return to live alone in her home, so arrangements are made for Naomi to move into a nursing home. Naomi becomes very depressed and withdrawn. The physician believes Naomi would benefit from an antidepressant medication. Which of the following is an example of an antidepressant that the physician may prescribe for Naomi?
    - a. Haloperidol (Haldol)
    - b. Tacrine (Cognex)
    - c. Sertraline (Zoloft)
    - d. Diazepam (Valium)

6. A 74-year-old exhibits more frequent memory loss and disorientation to time and place. The family tells the nurse that their loved one has been recently diagnosed with Alzheimer's disease. The nurse should know that the characteristics of this disease are:
    - a. Self-limiting.
    - b. An abrupt onset and a variable course.
    - c. Rapid functional decline in multiple cognitive areas.
    - d. Slow and insidious with a gradual and progressive loss of cognitive abilities.

7. The nurse working on an Alzheimer's disease unit should be aware that one of the first cognitive changes in a person diagnosed as having the disease would be:
    - a. Aphasia
    - b. Apraxia
    - c. Ataxia

- d. Memory disturbance

8. A 67-year-old female client is in the third stage of Alzheimer's disease. The nurse is aware that which of the following characteristics is indicative of this stage?
   - a. Forgetfulness is evident; confusion begins and interferes with work performance.
   - b. The individual loses the ability to perform activities of daily living independently.
   - c. Becomes mute and requires institutional care.
   - d. Apraxia progresses, may develop contractures, and aspiration of oral intake is common.

9. Many confused elderly persons smoke. The most appropriate nursing intervention would be to:
   - a. Restrict the number of cigarettes.
   - b. Restrict smoking privileges.
   - c. Monitor smoking periods.
   - d. Initiate a smoker's anonymous group.

10. Which of the following would be considered a *primary* dementia?
    - a. Dementia due to HIV disease
    - b. Dementia of the Alzheimer's type
    - c. Dementia due to cerebral trauma
    - d. Dementia related to nutritional deficiencies

CHAPTER 13. SUBSTANCE-RELATED DISORDERS

CHAPTER FOCUS

The focus of this chapter is on the physical and behavioral manifestations and personal and social consequences for the individual who abuses or is dependent on substances. Etiological implications are discussed, and the role of the nurse in the care of these clients is emphasized.

LEARNING OBJECTIVES

After reading this chapter, the student will be able to:
1. Define *abuse*, *dependence*, *intoxication*, and *withdrawal*.
2. Discuss etiological implications for substance-related disorders.
3. Identify symptomatology and use the information in assessment of clients with various substance-use disorders and substance-induced disorders.
4. Identify nursing diagnoses common to clients with substance-use disorders and substance-induced disorders, and select appropriate nursing interventions for each.
5. Identify topics for client and family teaching relevant to substance-use disorders and substance-induced disorders.
6. Describe relevant outcome criteria for evaluating nursing care of clients with substance-use disorders and substance-induced disorders.
7. Describe various modalities relevant to treatment of individuals with substance-use disorders and substance-induced disorders.

KEY TERMS

amphetamines
cannabis
opioids
phencyclidine
abuse
dependence
Wernicke's encephalopathy
Korsakoff's psychosis
ascites
esophageal varices
hepatic encephalopathy
Alcoholics Anonymous
disulfiram (Antabuse)
substitution therapy
detoxification
dual diagnosis

CHAPTER OUTLINE/LECTURE NOTES

I. Introduction
    A. Substance-related disorders are composed of two groups:
        1. Substance-use disorders
            a. **Abuse**
            b. **Dependence**
        2. Substance-induced disorders (Only intoxication and withdrawal are discussed in this chapter.)
            a. Intoxication
            b. Withdrawal
            c. Delirium
            d. Dementia
            e. Amnesia
            f. Psychosis
            g. Mood disorder
            h. Sexual dysfunction
            i. Sleep disorders
    B. Some illegal substances have achieved a degree of social acceptance by various subcultural groups within our society.

II. Substance-Use Disorders
    A. Substance abuse. *DSM-IV-TR* criteria for substance abuse:
        1. Recurrent substance use resulting in a failure to fulfill major role obligations at work, school, or home.
        2. Recurrent substance use in situations in which such use is physically hazardous.
        3. Recurrent substance-related legal problems.
        4. Continued substance use despite having persistent or recurrent social or interpersonal problems caused or exacerbated by the effects of the substance use.
    B. Substance dependence
        1. Physical dependence is manifested by the need for increasing amounts to produce the desired effects and a syndrome of withdrawal upon cessation.
        2. Psychological dependence exists when an individual believes that use of a substance is necessary to maintain an optimal state of personal well-being, interpersonal relations, or skill performance.
        3. *DSM-IV-TR* criteria for substance dependence include the following:
            a. Evidence of tolerance, as defined by either of the following:
                (1) A need for markedly increased amounts of the substance to achieve intoxication or desired effects.
                (2) Markedly diminished effect with continued use of the same amount of the substance.
            b. Evidence of withdrawal symptoms, as manifested by either of the following:
                (1) The characteristic withdrawal syndrome for the substance.

       (2) The same (or a closely related) substance is taken to relieve or avoid withdrawal symptoms.

    c. The substance is often taken in larger amounts or over a longer period than was intended.

    d. There is a persistent desire or multiple unsuccessful efforts to cut down or control substance use.

    e. A great deal of time is spent in activities necessary to obtain the substance, use the substance, or recover from its effects.

    f. Important social, occupational, or recreational activities are given up or reduced because of substance use.

    g. The substance use is continued despite knowledge of having a persistent or recurrent physical or psychological problem that is likely to have been caused or exacerbated by the substance.

III. Substance-Induced Disorders

    A. Substance intoxication. *DSM-IV-TR* criteria include:

      1. The development of a reversible substance-specific syndrome caused by recent ingestion of (or exposure to) a substance.

      2. Clinically significant maladaptive behavior or psychological changes that are due to the effect of the substance on the CNS and develop during or shortly after use of the substance.

      3. The symptoms are not due to a general medical condition and are not better accounted for by another mental disorder.

    B. Substance withdrawal. *DSM-IV-TR* criteria include:

      1. The development of a substance-specific syndrome caused by the cessation of (or reduction in) heavy and prolonged substance use.

      2. The substance-specific syndrome causes clinically significant distress or impairment in social, occupational, or other important areas of functioning.

      3. The symptoms are not due to a general medical condition and are not better accounted for by another mental disorder.

IV. Classes of Psychoactive Substances

    A. Alcohol

    B. **Amphetamines** and related substances

    C. Caffeine

    D. **Cannabis**

    E. Cocaine

    F. Hallucinogens

    G. Inhalants

    H. Nicotine

    I. **Opioids**

    J. **Phencyclidine** and related substances

    K. Sedatives, hypnotics, or anxiolytics

V. Etiological Implications

    A. Biological factors

      1. Genetics. Apparent hereditary factor, particularly with alcoholism.

2. Biochemical. Alcohol may produce morphine-like substances in the brain that are responsible for alcohol addiction.
  B. Psychological factors
    1. Developmental influences. May relate to severe ego impairment and disturbances in the sense of self.
    2. Personality factors. Certain personality traits have been suggested to play a part in both the development and maintenance of alcohol dependence. They include impulsivity, negative self-concept, weak ego, low social conformity, neuroticism, and introversion.
  C. Sociocultural factors
    1. Social learning. Children and adolescents are more likely to use substances if they have parents who provide a model for substance use. Use of substances may also be promoted within one's peer group.
    2. Conditioning. Pleasurable effects from substance use act as a positive reinforcement for their continued use.
    3. Cultural and ethnic influences. Some cultures are more prone to use of substances than others.
IV. Dynamics of Substance-Related Disorders
  A. Alcohol abuse and dependence
    1. A profile of the substance
    2. Historical aspects
    3. Patterns of use/abuse
      a. Phase I. The prealcoholic phase
      b. Phase II. The early alcoholic phase
      c. Phase III. The crucial phase
      d. Phase IV. The chronic phase
    4. Effects on the body
      a. Peripheral neuropathy
      b. Alcoholic myopathy
      c. **Wernicke's encephalopathy**
      d. **Korsakoff's psychosis**
      e. Alcoholic cardiomyopathy
      f. Esophagitis
      g. Gastritis
      h. Pancreatitis
      i. Alcoholic hepatitis
      j. Cirrhosis of the liver
        (1) Portal hypertension
        (2) **Ascites**
        (3) **Esophageal varices**
        (4) **Hepatic encephalopathy**
      k. Leukopenia
      l. Thrombocytopenia
      m. Sexual dysfunction
  B. Alcohol intoxication

    1. Occurs at blood alcohol levels between 100 and 200 mg/dl
C. Alcohol withdrawal
    1. Occurs within 4 to 12 hours of cessation of or reduction in heavy and prolonged alcohol use.
D. Sedative, hypnotic, or anxiolytic abuse and dependence
    1. A profile of the substance
        a. Barbiturates
        b. Nonbarbiturate hypnotics
        c. Antianxiety agents
    2. Historical aspects
    3. Patterns of use/abuse
    4. Effects on the body
        a. Effects on sleep and dreaming
        b. Respiratory depression
        c. Cardiovascular effects
        d. Renal function
        e. Hepatic effects
        f. Body temperature
        g. Sexual functioning
E. Sedative, hypnotic, or anxiolytic intoxication
    1. Intoxication with these CNS depressants can range from disinhibition and aggressiveness to coma and death (with increasing dosages of the drug).
F. Sedative, hypnotic, or anxiolytic withdrawal
    1. Onset of symptoms depends on the half-life of the drug from which the individual is withdrawing.
    2. Severe withdrawal from CNS depressants can be life threatening.
G. CNS stimulant abuse and dependence
    1. A profile of the substance
        a. Amphetamines
        b. Nonamphetamine stimulants
        c. Cocaine
        d. Caffeine
        e. Nicotine
    2. Historical aspects
    3. Patterns of use/abuse
    4. Effects on the body
        a. CNS effects
        b. Cardiovascular/pulmonary effects
        c. Gastrointestinal and renal effects
        d. Sexual functioning
H. CNS stimulant intoxication
    1. Amphetamine and cocaine intoxication produces euphoria, impaired judgment, confusion, changes in vital signs (even coma or death, depending on amount consumed).

2. Intoxication from caffeine usually occurs following consumption in excess of 250 mg. Restlessness and insomnia are the most common symptoms.

I. CNS stimulant withdrawal
   1. Withdrawal from amphetamines and cocaine may include dysphoria, fatigue, sleep disturbances, and increased appetite.
   2. Withdrawal from caffeine may include headache, fatigue, anxiety, and nausea and vomiting.
   3. Withdrawal from nicotine may include dysphoria, anxiety, difficulty concentrating, restlessness, and increased appetite.

J. Inhalant abuse and dependence
   1. A profile of the substance
      a. Aliphatic and aromatic hydrocarbons
      b. Examples include gasoline, varnish remover, lighter fluid, airplane glue, rubber cement, cleaning fluid, spray paint, shoe conditioner, and typewriter correction fluid
   2. Patterns of use/abuse
   3. Effects on the body
      a. CNS effects
      b. Respiratory effects
      c. GI effects
      d. Renal system effects

K. Inhalant intoxication
   1. The *DSM-IV-TR* defines inhalant intoxication as "clinically significant maladaptive behavioral or psychological changes that develop during, or shortly after, use of or exposure to volatile inhalants."
   2. Symptoms may include dizziness, nystagmus, incoordination, slurred speech, unsteady gait, lethargy, depressed reflexes, psychomotor retardation, tremor, generalized muscle weakness, blurred vision or diplopia, stupor or coma, or euphoria.

L. Opioid abuse and dependence
   1. A profile of the substance
      a. Opioids of natural origin
      b. Opioid derivatives
      c. Synthetic opiate-like drugs
   2. Historical aspects
   3. Patterns of use/abuse
   4. Effects on the body
      a. CNS effects
      b. GI effects
      c. Cardiovascular effects
      d. Sexual functioning

M. Opioid intoxication
   1. Symptoms are consistent with the half-life of most opioid drugs and usually last for several hours.
   2. Severe opioid intoxication can lead to respiratory depression, coma, and death.

N. Opioid withdrawal
1. Symptoms occur within 6 to 24 hours after the last dose, peak within 1 to 3 days, and gradually subside over a period of 5 to 7 days (these might differ according to drug half-life).
O. Hallucinogen abuse and dependence
1. A profile of the substance
a. Naturally-occurring hallucinogens
(1) Mescaline
(2) Psilocybin and psilocyn
(3) Ololiugui
b. Synthetic compounds
(1) LSD
(2) Dimethyltryptamine
(3) 2,5-dimethoxy-4-methamphetamine (STP)
(4) Phencyclidine hydrochloride (PCP)
(5) Designer drugs
2. Historical aspects
3. Patterns of use/abuse
4. Effects on the body
P. Hallucinogen intoxication
1. Occurs within minutes to a few hours after using the drug.
2. Symptoms include perceptual alteration, depersonalization, derealization, tachycardia, and palpitations. Symptoms of PCP intoxication also include belligerence and assaultiveness and may proceed to seizures or coma.
Q. Cannabis abuse and dependence
1. A profile of the substance
a. Marijuana
b. Hashish
2. Historical aspects
3. Patterns of use/abuse
4. Effects on the body
a. Cardiovascular effects
b. Respiratory effects
c. Reproductive effects
d. CNS effects
e. Sexual functioning
R. Cannabis intoxication
1. Symptoms include impaired motor coordination, euphoria, anxiety, a sensation of slowed time, and impaired judgment.
2. Impairment of motor skills lasts for 8 to 12 hours.
VII. Application of the Nursing Process
A. Nurse must begin relationship development with a substance abuser by examining their own attitudes and drinking habits.
B. Various assessment tools are available for determining the extent of a client's problem with substances.

1. Drug history and assessment
2. Michigan Alcoholism Screening Test (MAST)
3. CAGE Questionnaire

C. **Dual diagnosis**
1. Determination is made that the client has a substance disorder co-existing with mental illness.
2. Client is assigned to a special program that targets both problems.

D. Nursing diagnoses are formulated from the data gathered during the assessment phase. Outcome criteria are established for each.

E. Nursing intervention for the client with substance use disorder is aimed at acceptance of use of substances as a problem, acceptance of personal responsibility for use of substances, identification of more adaptive coping strategies, and restoration of nutritional status.

F. Client/family education.

G. Evaluation of care is based on achievement of the outcome criteria.

VIII. Treatment Modalities for Substance-Related Disorders

A. **Alcoholics Anonymous**

B. Various support groups are patterned after Alcoholics Anonymous, but for individuals with problems with other substances.

C. Pharmacotherapy:
1. **Disulfiram (Antabuse).**
2. Other medications for treatment of alcoholism.

D. Counseling

E. Group Therapy

F. Psychopharmacology for Substance Intoxication and Substance Withdrawal

IX. Summary

X. Critical Thinking Exercise

XI. Review Questions

ANSWERS TO CRITICAL THINKING EXERCISE

1. Risk for suicide.
2. Suicide precautions. Decrease environmental stimuli. Let her sleep as much as she wants. Provide adequate diet to restore nutrition.
3. To help her recognize the correlation between taking the drugs and the problems she is having in her life.

LEARNING ACTIVITY

SYMPTOMS ASSOCIATED WITH PSYCHOACTIVE SUBSTANCES

Fill in the spaces provided with the most common examples and symptoms of substance-related disorders of which the nurse should be aware.

Drugs	Symptoms of Use	Symptoms of Intoxication	Symptoms of Withdrawal
CNS Depressants Examples:			
CNS Stimulants Examples:			
Opioids Examples:			
Hallucinogens Examples:			
Cannabinols Examples:			
Inhalants Examples:			

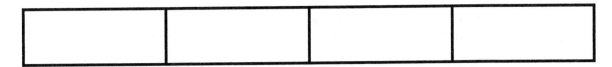

CASE STUDIES FOR USE WITH STUDENT LEARNING

Case Study: Cocaine Intoxication

Lance, age 18, is brought into the emergency department by the police. He was first taken to the Police Department after being picked up with a friend trying to break into a house to steal money to buy more cocaine. However, Lance's physical condition deteriorated (nausea, vomiting, tremors). When he experienced a seizure, the police brought him to the ED. His blood pressure and heart rate are elevated. The police state that Lance's friend reported to them that Lance has been binging on cocaine for several days. When they ran out of the drug, they decided to steal money to buy more. After a great deal of prodding, the friend gave the police the name of Lance's mother, who was called by the ED nurse. She appeared to be somewhat agitated about being awakened in the middle of the night. She reported that she hasn't been able to control her son's behavior for a number of years now. He started drinking and hanging out with an older crowd when he was about 13 years old. Lance's father left the home when Lance was 4 years old, and no one has heard from him since. Lance's mother works as a waitress, when she can get work. She admits that she drinks too much, but states, "It's the only way I can deal with all my problems." The ED physician admits Lance to the psychiatric unit for cocaine **detoxification**. Design a nursing care plan for Lance.

Case Study: Alcohol Withdrawal Delirium

Sam, a 45-year-old construction worker, is brought into the emergency department by his brother, John. Sam is incoherent, disoriented, tremulous, and shifts in and out of consciousness. At times he makes comments about bugs crawling on his skin. Sam has lived alone for 6 years since his wife died of cancer. They had no children. John brought Sam to the ED after receiving a call from Sam's neighbor who reported seeing Sam weaving in and out of traffic on the street in front of their houses. John reports that he sees Sam infrequently, but believes that Sam drinks whiskey on a daily basis, and probably has increased the amount he drinks over the last few years. Sam lost his job a few weeks ago and has been drinking heavily ever since. John postulates that Sam ran out of whiskey a few days ago and hasn't had money to buy more. John could find no food or alcohol in the house when he went to pick Sam up. The physician admits Sam to the psychiatric unit with a diagnosis of Alcohol Withdrawal Delirium. Lorazepam (Ativan) is ordered on a scheduled and p.r.n. basis. Design a nursing care plan for Sam.

Case Study: Alcohol Dependence

After being treated for Alcohol Withdrawal, Sam has been told by his physician that he has alcoholic cardiomyopathy and that if he does not abstain from alcohol, he will die.

Sam decides to go into a rehabilitation program for alcohol dependence. Design a nursing care plan for Sam during the beginning phase of his rehabilitation.

TEST QUESTIONS

Situation: Michael, a 47-year-old salesman, is brought to the emergency department at midnight by the police because of aggressive, disinhibited behavior, slurred speech, and impaired motor coordination. His blood alcohol level is found to be 347 mg/dl. He is admitted to the Alcohol and Drug Treatment Unit for detoxification.

1. At what minimum level of alcohol in the blood is an individual considered to be intoxicated?
    - a. 50 mg/dl
  - • b. 100 mg/dl
    - c. 200 mg/dl
    - d. 300 mg/dl

2. Michael's wife is notified, and she reports to the admitting nurse that Michael's drinking has increased over the last several years. Michael has lately been drinking a pint of bourbon a day, mostly in the evening, but sometimes also during the day. "He usually just comes home from work and drinks until he passes out." She stated that yesterday Michael's boss told him if he didn't increase his sales, he would be fired. Michael started drinking in the early afternoon and drank continuously into the night. She didn't know what time he left the house. It is now 2:00 A.M. When might the nurse expect withdrawal symptoms to begin?
  - • a. Around 4:00 to 6:00 A.M.
    - b. Around 2:00 P.M.
    - c. In 2 to 3 days
    - d. Around 4:00 to 6:00 P.M.

3. For what initial withdrawal symptoms should the nurse be on the alert?
    - a. Suicidal ideation, increased appetite
    - b. Lacrimation, rhinorrhea, piloerection
  - • c. Tremors, tachycardia, sweating
    - d. Belligerence, assaultiveness

4. What would be the expected treatment for Michael as he withdraws from alcohol?
    - a. Tricyclic antidepressants
    - b. A long-acting barbiturate, such as phenobarbital
    - c. Alcohol deterrent therapy, such as disulfiram

- d. Substitution therapy with chlordiazepoxide

5. The physician also orders daily administration of Thiamine for Michael. What is the rationale behind this order?
    a. To restore nutritional balance
    b. To prevent pancreatitis
    c. To prevent alcoholic hepatitis
- d. To prevent Wernicke's encephalopathy

6. Symptoms of the correct answer to the previous question include:
    a. Peripheral neuropathy and pain.
    b. Epigastric pain and nausea/vomiting.
- c. Diplopia, ataxia, somnolence.
    d. Inflammation and necrosis of the liver.

7. Although Michael denies that he is an alcoholic, the nurse encourages him to seek rehabilitative treatment. The nurse understands that for Michael to be successful in treatment, he must first:
    a. Identify someone to whom he can go for support.
    b. Give up all his old drinking buddies.
    c. Understand the dynamics of alcohol on the body.
- d. Correlate life problems to his drinking of alcohol.

General questions related to substance-related disorders:

8. Methadone may be administered to an individual in opioid withdrawal to:
    a. Augment the addict's craving for narcotics.
- b. Provide a longer-acting narcotic that is a substitute for heroin.
    c. Administer a legally controlled drug.
    d. Improve psychological well-being and family and social functioning.

9. A drug commonly used for opioid intoxication is:
    a. Benztropine (Cogentin).
    b. Methohexital sodium (Brevital).
- c. Nalorphine (Nalline).
    d. Chlordiazepoxide (Librium).

10. A nurse assessing a client in cannabis intoxication might expect to see which of the following symptoms:

- a. Euphoria, conjunctival redness, and increased appetite.
- b. Belligerence, assaultiveness, and blurred vision.
- c. Elevated blood pressure, grandiosity, nausea, and vomiting.
- d. Decreased respiratory rate, pinpoint pupils, and muscle rigidity.

CHAPTER 14. SCHIZOPHRENIA AND OTHER PSYCHOTIC DISORDERS

CHAPTER FOCUS

The focus of this chapter is on nursing care of the client with psychotic disorders. Etiological implications and symptomatology are explored, and nursing care is presented in the context of the nursing process. Medical treatment modalities are also discussed.

LEARNING OBJECTIVES

After reading this chapter, the student will be able to:
1. Discuss the concepts of schizophrenia and related psychotic disorders.
2. Identify etiological implications in the development of these disorders.
3. Describe various types of schizophrenia and related psychotic disorders.
4. Identify symptomatology associated with these disorders and use this information in client assessment.
5. Formulate nursing diagnoses and goals of care for clients with schizophrenia and other psychotic disorders.
6. Identify topics for client and family teaching relevant to schizophrenia and other psychotic disorders.
7. Describe appropriate nursing interventions for behaviors associated with these disorders.
8. Describe relevant criteria for evaluating nursing care of clients with schizophrenia and related psychotic disorders.
9. Discuss various modalities relevant to treatment of schizophrenia and related psychotic disorders.

KEY TERMS

delusions	circumstantiality
hallucinations	tangentiality
illusion	perseveration
echolalia	catatonic
paranoia	autism
echopraxia	waxy flexibility
religiosity	anhedonia
magical thinking	associative looseness
neuroleptic	social skills training
neologism	clang association
word salad	

CHAPTER OUTLINE/LECTURE NOTES

I. Introduction
   A. The word *schizophrenia* is derived from the Greek words *skhizo* (split) and *phren* (mind).
   B. Schizophrenia is probably caused by a combination of factors, including genetic predisposition, biochemical dysfunction, and psychosocial stress.
   C. Schizophrenia requires treatment that is comprehensive and is presented in a multidisciplinary effort.
   D. Schizophrenia probably causes more lengthy hospitalizations, more chaos in family life, more exorbitant costs to individuals and governments, and more fears than any other mental illness.

II. Nature of the Disorder
   A. Schizophrenia results in disturbances in thought processes, perception, and affect.
   B. There is severe deterioration of social and occupational functioning.
   C. Approximately 1 percent of the population will develop schizophrenia over the course of a lifetime.
   D. The premorbid behavior of an individual with schizophrenia can be viewed in four phases.
      1. Phase I. The schizoid personality. Indifferent, cold, and aloof, these individuals are loners. They do not enjoy close relationships with others.
      2. Phase II. The prodromal phase. In this phase, the individuals are socially withdrawn, and have behavior that is peculiar or eccentric. Role functioning is impaired, personal hygiene is neglected, and disturbances exist in communication, ideation, and perception.
      3. Phase III. Schizophrenia. In the active phase of the disorder, psychotic symptoms are prominent. These include **delusions**, **hallucinations**, and impairment in work, social relations, and self-care.
      4. Phase IV. Residual phase. Symptoms similar to the prodromal phase, with flat affect and impairment in role functioning being prominent.

III. Etiological Implications
   A. Biological influences
      1. Genetics. A growing body of knowledge indicates that genetics plays an important role in the development of schizophrenia.
      2. Biochemical influences. One theory suggests that schizophrenia may be caused by an excess of dopamine-dependent neuronal activity in the brain. Abnormalities in the neurotransmitters norepinephrine, serotonin, acetylcholine, and gamma-aminobutyric acid have also been suggested.
      3. Physiological influences. Several physiological factors have been implicated, including viral infection, brain abnormalities, and histological changes in the brain. Various physical conditions, such as epilepsy, systemic lupus erythematosus, myxedema, Parkinsonism, and Wilson's disease, have also been implicated.
   B. Psychological influences. Purely psychological factors are being questioned at this time. Researchers in the last decade are focusing their studies more in terms of schizophrenia as a brain disorder. The psychological theories probably developed early on out of a lack of information related to a biological connection.

C. Environmental influences
   1. Sociocultural factors. Lower socioeconomic status has been linked to the development of schizophrenia.
   2. Stressful life events have been associated with the onset of schizophrenic symptoms. Responses vary according to the number and severity of life events and the degree of vulnerability to the impact of the life event.
D. Theoretical integration. Schizophrenia is most likely the result of a combination of biological, psychological, and environmental influences on an individual who is vulnerable to the illness.

IV. Types of Schizophrenia and Other Psychotic Disorders
  A. Disorganized schizophrenia. Chronic variety with flat or inappropriate affect. Silliness and incongruous giggling is common. Behavior is bizarre, and social interaction is impaired.
  B. **Catatonic** schizophrenia
    1. Catatonic stupor. Characterized by extreme psychomotor retardation. The individual is usually mute. Posturing is common.
    2. Catatonic excitement. Extreme psychomotor agitation. Purposeless movements that must be curtailed to prevent injury to the client or others.
  C. Paranoid schizophrenia. Characterized by paranoid delusions. Client may be argumentative, hostile, and aggressive.
  D. Undifferentiated schizophrenia. Bizarre behavior that does not meet the criteria outlined for the other types of schizophrenia, or may meet the criteria for more than one type. Delusions and hallucinations are prominent.
  E. Residual schizophrenia. This category is used for the individual who has a history of at least one episode of schizophrenia with prominent psychotic symptoms. Also known as ambulatory schizophrenia, this is the stage that follows an acute episode.
  F. Schizoaffective disorder. Schizophrenic symptoms accompanied by a strong element of symptomatology associated with the mood disorders, either mania or depression.
  G. Brief psychotic disorder. Sudden onset of psychotic symptoms following a severe psychosocial stressor. Symptoms last less than 1 month, and the individual returns to the full premorbid level of functioning.
  H. Schizophreniform disorder. Same symptoms as schizophrenia with the exception that the duration of the disorder has been at least 1 month but less than 6 months.
  I. Delusional disorder. The existence of prominent, nonbizarre delusions.
    1. Erotomanic type. The individual believes that someone, usually of a higher status, is in love with him or her.
    2. Grandiose type. Irrational ideas regarding own worth, talent, knowledge, or power.
    3. Jealous type. Irrational idea that the person's sexual partner is unfaithful.
    4. Persecutory type. The individual believes he or she is being malevolently treated in some way.
    5. Somatic type. The individual has an irrational belief that he or she has some physical defect, disorder, or disease.

J. Shared psychotic disorder. A delusional system develops in a second person as a result of a close relationship with another person who already has a psychotic disorder with prominent delusions. Also called *folie à deux*.

K. Psychotic disorder due to a general medical dondition. Symptoms of this disorder include prominent hallucinations and delusions that can be directly attributed to a general medical condition.

L. Substance-induced psychotic disorder. The presence of prominent hallucinations and delusions that are judged to be directly attributable to the physiological effects of a substance.

V. Application of the Nursing Process

A. Background assessment data

1. Content of Thought
   a. Delusions: false personal beliefs
   b. **Religiosity**: excessive demonstration of obsession with religious ideas and behavior
   c. **Paranoia**: extreme suspiciousness of others
   d. **Magical thinking**: the idea that if one thinks something it will be true

2. Form of thought
   a. **Associative looseness**: shift of ideas from one topic to another
   b. **Neologisms**: made-up words that have meaning only to the individual who invents them
   c. Concrete thinking: literal interpretations of the environment
   d. **Clang associations**: choice of words is governed by sound (often rhyming)
   e. **Word salad**: a group of words put together in a random fashion
   f. **Circumstantiality**: a delay in reaching the point of a communication due to unnecessary and tedious details
   g. **Tangentiality**: inability to get to point of communication due to introduction of many new topics
   h. Mutism: inability or refusal to speak
   i. **Perseveration**: persistent repetition of the same word or idea in response to different questions

3. Perception: the interpretation of stimuli through the senses
   a. Hallucinations: false sensory perceptions not associated with real external stimuli
   b. **Illusions**: misperceptions of real external stimuli

4. Affect: emotional tone
   a. Inappropriate affect: emotions that are incongruent with the circumstances
   b. Bland or flat affect: weak emotional tone
   c. Apathy: disinterest in the environment

5. Sense of self: the uniqueness and individuality a person feels
   a. **Echolalia**: repeating words that are heard
   b. **Echopraxia**: repeating movements that are observed

c. Identification and imitation: taking on the form of behavior one observes in another

d. Depersonalization: feelings of unreality

6. Volition: impairment in the ability to initiate goal-directed activity

   a. Emotional ambivalence: the coexistence of opposite emotions toward the same object

7. Impaired interpersonal functioning and relationship to the external world

   a. **Autism**: the focus inward on a fantasy world while distorting or excluding the external environment

   b. Deteriorated appearance: personal grooming and self-care activities are impaired

8. Psychomotor behavior

   a. Anergia: a deficiency of energy

   b. **Waxy flexibility**: passive yielding of all moveable parts of the body to any efforts made at placing them in certain positions

   c. Posturing: voluntary assumption of inappropriate or bizarre postures

   d. Pacing and rocking: pacing back and forth and rocking of the body

9. Associated features

   a. **Anhedonia**: inability to experience pleasure

   b. Regression: retreating to an earlier level of development

10. Positive and negative symptoms

    a. Positive symptoms reflect an excess or distortion of normal functions, such as disorganized thinking, and are thought to have a relatively good response to treatment.

    b. Negative symptoms reflect a diminution or loss of normal functions, such as diminished emotional expression and apathy, and are less likely than the positive symptoms to respond to treatment.

B. Nursing diagnosis/outcome identification

   1. Nursing diagnoses

      a. Alteration in thought processes

      b. Sensory-perceptual alteration: audio/visual

      c. Social isolation

      d. Risk for violence: self or others

      e. Impaired verbal communication

      f. Self-care deficit

      g. Ineffective family coping: disabling

      h. Altered health maintenance

      i. Impaired home-maintenance management

   2. Outcome criteria

C. Planning/implementation

   1. Care plan for the client with schizophrenia

D. Client/family education

E. Evaluation

   1. Reassessment data on which to base the effectiveness of nursing actions

VI. Treatment Modalities for Schizophrenia and Other Psychotic Disorders

A. Psychological treatments
   1. Individual psychotherapy. Long-term therapeutic approach; difficult because of client's impairment in interpersonal functioning.
   2. Group therapy. Some success if occurring over the long-term course of the illness; less successful in acute treatment.
   3. Behavior therapy. Chief drawback has been the inability to generalize to the community setting once the client has been discharged from the hospital.
   4. **Social skills training**. The use of role play to teach client appropriate eye contact, interpersonal skills, voice intonation, posture, and so forth. The aim is improvement in relationship development
B. Social treatment
   1. Milieu therapy. Best if used in conjunction with psychopharmacology
   2. Family therapy. Aimed at helping family members cope with the long-term effects of the illness
C. Organic treatment
   1. Psychopharmacology
      a. Antipsychotics. Used to decrease agitation and psychotic symptoms.
      b. Antiparkinsonian agents. Used to counteract the extrapyramidal symptoms associated with antipsychotic medications.
      c. Others. Reserpine, lithium carbonate, carbamazepine, valium, and propranolol have been used with mixed results.
VII. Summary
VIII. Critical Thinking Exercise
IX. Review Questions

ANSWERS TO CRITICAL THINKING EXERCISE

1. Possible command hallucinations
2. Alteration in sensory-perception: auditory
3. Decrease Sara's anxiety and establish trust

CASE STUDY FOR USE WITH STUDENT LEARNING

Case Study: Paranoid Schizophrenia

Caroline, age 22, was diagnosed with paranoid schizophrenia at age 19. She led a relatively normal life during grade school and high school years. She left her parents at age 17 to attend a college somewhat distant to her home. She apparently had no problems during her first year, but when she returned for Thanksgiving break during her second year, her parents noticed a distancing about her. She spent a lot of time alone, was irritable, and had begun chain smoking and drinking alcohol. She failed two courses that fall and was placed on probation. When she went back to school in the spring, her former roommate refused to stay with her, saying, "She acts so crazy sometimes. She talks out of her head, and I'm afraid of her." In late February, Caroline's parents got a call from the Dean of Students who related that the campus police had to be called to Caroline's room to quiet her. She had been "yelling and screaming" and no one could understand what it had been all about. She had apparently really frightened the other students in the dormitory. These bizarre behaviors continued, and during spring break in March, Caroline's parents moved her home and made an appointment with a psychiatrist for an evaluation. During the assessment, Caroline's thought processes were loose, vague, and often circumstantial. She exhibited behaviors that suggested auditory hallucinations (stopping mid-sentence and "cocking" her head to the side as if listening), although when questioned about whether or not she heard voices, she denied it. Paranoid delusional thinking was evident. She made statements such as, "There is no one I can trust at that college. Every student in that dorm has been told to keep an eye on me. They all know I am too smart to be there, so they will do what they can to make me fail. If I pass, then everyone else fails." She also expressed somatic delusions: "I'm pregnant, you know. It will be a virgin birth. That's another reason the college kids are out to get me. They are so jealous! I am the chosen one." Since that time, she has been on several antipsychotic medications (chlorpromazine, clozapine, and risperidone), each with only minimal success, and which she would eventually quit taking altogether. She currently lives at home with her parents, who are beside themselves with concern and frustration. The psychiatrist has admitted Caroline to the hospital at this time to evaluate her behavior and to begin her on a trial of fluphenazine decanoate, which will eventually be administered only every 3 weeks by IM injection, in an effort to encourage increased medication compliance on Caroline's part. Design a nursing care plan for Caroline during this hospital admission.

LEARNING ACTIVITIES

I. Behaviors Associated with Schizophrenia

_____ 1. Autism	a. Kneels to pray in front of water fountain; prays during group therapy and during other group activities.
_____ 2. Mutism	b. Refuses to eat food that comes on tray, stating, "They are trying to poison me."
_____ 3. Hallucination	c. "When I get out of the hospital I'm going to buy me a sprongle."
_____ 4. Persecutory delusion	d. Does not talk.
_____ 5. Word salad	e. Keeps arm in position nurse left it after taking blood pressure. Assumes this position for hours.
_____ 6. Religiosity	f. "When I speak, presidents and kings listen."
_____ 7. Associative looseness	g. A withdrawal inward into one's own fantasy world.
_____ 8. Inappropriate affect	h. "I'm going to the circus. Jesus is God. The police are playing for keeps."

_____ 9. Paranoia

i. "We can't close the drapes, for if we do, the sun won't shine.

_____ 10. Magical thinking

j. "Test, test, this is a test. I do not jest; we get no rest."

_____ 11. Neologism

k. Laughs when told that his or her mother has just died.

_____ 12. Clang association

l. In response to stressful situation, begins to suck thumb and soils clothing.

_____ 13. Waxy flexibility

m. "Get by for anyone just to answer fortune cookies."

_____ 14. Regression

n. "If the FBI finds me here, I'll never get out alive."

_____ 15. Delusion of grandeur

o. Stops talking in mid-sentence, tilts head to side, and listens.

II. Case Study

Read the following case study and fill in the blanks with the description of the information that is underlined and numbered in the text. The first is completed as an example.

Situation: Sandra is a 37-year-old woman who was picked up by the police after she ran away from her parents' home. Sandra has a history of paranoid schizophrenia for 17 years. She has had numerous hospitalizations.

The police were called when Sandra began wandering through a local park and screaming at everyone, "I know you are possessed by the devil!" During her initial interview, she is <u>very guarded and suspicious of the nurse</u> (1). <u>"I can read your mind, you know."</u> (2).

(1)_____paranoia_____

(2)_____

Sandra is assigned to a room and oriented to the unit. At 5:00 P.M., the nurse says to Sandra, "Sandra, it's time for dinner." <u>Sandra responds, "Time for dinner; time for dinner; time for dinner."</u>(3)

(3)_____

The nurse notices that <u>each time she wipes her mouth with her napkin at dinner, Sandra does the same.</u>(4)

(4)_____

Sandra's mother reports that Sandra stopped taking her medicine about a month ago, stating, <u>"When you don't have a brain,</u> (5) you don't need brain medicine." Shortly afterward, she became totally despondent, <u>taking no pleasure in activities she had always found enjoyable.</u>(6) She stayed in her room, sitting on her bed <u>moving back and forth in a slow, rhythmic fashion.</u>(7) Sometimes she would not even get up to go to the bathroom, <u>instead soiling herself in an infantile manner.</u>(8)

(5)_____

(6)_____

(7)_____

(8)_____

She seemed to experience a total <u>lack of energy for usual activities of daily living.</u>(9) On the unit, Sandra <u>appears disinterested in everything around her.</u>(10) She sits alone, <u>talking and laughing to herself.</u>(11) At one point she hears a laugh track on TV and states, <u>"They're laughing at me. I know they are."</u> (12)

(9)_____

(10)_____

(11)_____

(12)_____

Sandra's anxiety level starts to rise. She begins to pace the floor. Her agitation increases and she finally picks up a chair and hurls it toward the nurses' station, yelling, "The devil says all blonds must be annihilated!"

a. What would be Sandra's priority nursing diagnosis?

b. What medication would you expect the physician to order for Sandra?

c. For what adverse effects would you be on the alert with this drug?

d. In what developmental stage (Erikson) would you place Sandra? Why?

e. Theoretically, in what developmental stage *should* she be?

TEST QUESTIONS

Situation: Frankie, a 20-year-old college student, seemed "different" when he was home for Thanksgiving. His thinking was somewhat disorganized, and he was convinced that a fellow student was spreading untruths about him. After arriving home for the Christmas break, he stopped bathing and isolated himself in his room, often staying up all night and then sleeping most of the following day. He complained of voices whispering his name.

In April, Frankie's parents receive a call from the Dean of Students at Frankie's college. He tells them that Frankie has quit attending classes. He stays in his room all of the time, and often will not let his roommate enter. He yells accusations at his roommate and other students, believing that they are conspiring against him. Last night, he charged after his roommate with a knife in his hands. He was taken to the local hospital by the police and was admitted to the psychiatric unit. The psychiatrist has diagnosed Frankie with paranoid schizophrenia.

1. Based on the above information, what *initial* nursing diagnosis would the nurse make?
   a. Risk for self-directed violence
   b. Sensory-perceptual alteration
   - c. Risk for other-directed violence
   d. Altered thought processes

2. Based on background knowledge, in what stage of development would the nurse place Frankie?
   - a. Trust versus mistrust
   b. Autonomy versus shame and doubt
   c. Identity versus role confusion
   d. Intimacy versus isolation

3. Because of his developmental level, what must be an *initial* intervention for the nurse?
   - a. Allowing Frankie to take charge of his self-care independently
   - b. Putting Frankie in the first group therapy session with an opening
   - c. Helping Frankie decide where he wants to go in his life from here
   - • d. Helping Frankie decrease his anxiety and establish trust

4. The physician orders 100 mg chlorpromazine (Thorazine) b.i.d. and 2 mg benztropine (Cogentin) b.i.d., p.r.n. Rationale for the chlorpromazine order is:
   - a. To ensure that Frankie can get enough sleep.
   - • b. To reduce psychotic symptoms.
   - c. To decrease Frankie's aggressiveness.
   - d. To prevent tardive dyskinesia.

5. Under what circumstances would the nurse administer a dose of p.r.n. Cogentin?
   - a. When Frankie becomes aggressive
   - b. To calm Frankie down before bedtime
   - • c. When Frankie exhibits tremors and shuffling gait
   - d. When Frankie complains of constipation

6. Frankie says to the nurse, "My roommate was plotting with others to have me killed!" The most appropriate response by the nurse would be:
   - • a. "I find that hard to believe, Frankie."
   - b. "What would make you think such a thing?"
   - c. "No one was trying to kill you, Frankie."
   - d. "I might feel the same way if you came after *me* with a knife!"

7. The nurse notices that Frankie is stopping in midsentence when they are talking. He tilts his head to the side as if listening to something. The most appropriate intervention by the nurse would be:
   - a. Call and report the behavior to the physician.
   - b. Give Frankie a p.r.n. dose of benztropine.
   - • c. Say to Frankie, "What are the voices saying to you, Frankie?"
   - d. Say to Frankie, "Well, I see you are distracted right now. We'll talk more later."

8. John, who is admitted with undifferentiated schizophrenia, approaches the nurse and says, "I'm Jesus Christ and I'm here to forgive your sins." The most therapeutic response to the client at this time would be:
    - a. I understand that you think you are Jesus Christ, but I don't believe that you are."
    - b. "I'm your nurse for the evening shift today. Why don't we sit in the day room, and we can talk about why you are here.
    - c. "You know that you are not Jesus Christ, and if you continue to say that you are, the other clients may not want to associate with you."
    - d. "I'll have to report this to your physician. He'll be very interested in hearing about this."

9. John gets fluphenazine 2 mg b.i.d. John's doctor also prescribes benztropine p.r.n. for John. Why would the physician most likely elect to prescribe the benztropine p.r.n. rather than on a routinely scheduled basis?
    - a. Because it commonly causes extrapyramidal side effects
    - b. To prevent compounded anticholinergic side effects with the antipsychotic medication
    - c. Because of the adverse cardiovascular side effects associated with benztropine
    - d. Because it is highly unlikely that John will even need the benztropine

10. John says to the nurse, "The ball will fall in the stall. Call me at the mall." The nurse assesses John's verbalizations as:
    - a. Neologisms.
    - b. Circumstantiality.
    - c. Clang associations.
    - d. Magical thinking.

11. What would be the nurse's best response to the statement made by John in question #10?
    - a. "You are not making any sense, John."
    - b. "Are you telling me that you want to go to the mall, John?"
    - c. "How do you expect me to help you, John, if you keep talking like that?"
    - d. "I don't understand what you mean, John. Please explain it to me."

CHAPTER 15. MOOD DISORDERS

CHAPTER FOCUS

The focus of this chapter is on nursing care of the client with mood disorders (depression or mania). Etiological implications and symptomatology are explored, and nursing care is presented in the context of the six steps of the nursing process. Medical treatment modalities are also discussed.

LEARNING OBJECTIVES

After reading this chapter, the student will be able to:
1. Recount historical perspectives of mood disorders.
2. Discuss epidemiological statistics related to mood disorders.
3. Describe various types of mood disorders.
4. Identify etiological implications in the development of mood disorders.
5. Discuss implications of depression related to developmental stages.
6. Identify symptomatology associated with mood disorders and use this information in client assessment.
7. Formulate nursing diagnoses and goals of care for clients with mood disorders.
8. Identify topics for client and family teaching relevant to mood disorders.
9. Describe appropriate nursing interventions for behaviors associated with mood disorders.
10. Describe relevant criteria for evaluating nursing care of clients with mood disorders.
11. Discuss various modalities relevant to treatment of mood disorders.

KEY TERMS

electroconvulsive therapy
bipolar disorder
cognitive therapy
cyclothymic disorder
psychomotor retardation
delirious mania
premenstrual dysphoric disorder
postpartum depression
hypomania
mania
melancholia
mood

CHAPTER OUTLINE/LECTURE NOTES

I.   Introduction

A. Depression is the oldest and most frequently described psychiatric illness.
B. Transient symptoms are normal, healthy responses to everyday disappointments in life.
C. Pathological depression occurs when adaptation is ineffective.
D. Various medical treatment modalities are explored.

II. Historical Perspective
A. Many ancient cultures have believed in the supernatural or divine origin of depression and **mania**.
B. Hippocrates believed that **melancholia** was caused by an excess of black bile, a heavily toxic substance produced in the spleen or intestine, which affected the brain.
C. Various other theories were espoused regarding the etiology of depression. It was described as the result of obstruction of vital air circulation, excessive brooding, or helpless situations beyond the client's control.
D. Nineteenth-century definitions of mania narrowed it down to a disorder of affect and action.
E. The perspectives of 20th century theorists lend support to the notion of multiple causation in the development of **mood** disorders.

III. Epidemiology
A. Ten to 14 million Americans are afflicted with some form of major affective disorder.
B. Gender. Depression is more prevalent in women than it is in men. **Bipolar disorder** is roughly equal.
C. Age. Depression is more common in young women and has a tendency to decrease with age. The opposite is true with men. Studies regarding bipolar disorder suggest that the median age at onset of bipolar disorder is 18 years in men and 20 years in women.
D. Social class. There is an inverse relationship between social class and report of depressive symptoms. The opposite is true with bipolar disorder.
E. Race. No consistent relationship between race and affective disorder has been reported.
F. Marital status. Single and divorced persons are more likely to experience depression than married persons.
G. Seasonality. Affective disorders are more prevalent in the spring and in the fall.

IV. Types of Mood Disorders
A. Depressive disorders
   1. Major depressive disorder
      a. Single episode or recurrent
      b. Mild, moderate, or severe
      c. With psychotic features
      d. With catatonic features
      e. With melancholic features
      f. Chronic
      g. With seasonal pattern
      h. With postpartum onset

2. Dysthymic disorder
   a. Early onset
   b. Late onset
3. **Premenstrual dysphoric disorder**
B. Bipolar disorders
   1. Bipolar I disorder
   2. Bipolar II disorder
   3. **Cyclothymic disorder**
C. Other mood disorders
   1. Mood disorder due to a general medical condition
   2. Substance-induced mood disorder
V. Depressive disorders
   A. Etiological implications
      1. Biological theories
         a. Genetics. Hereditary factor may be involved.
         b. Biochemical influences. Deficiency of norepinephrine, serotonin, and dopamine have been implicated.
         c. Neuroendocrine disturbances
            (1) Possible failure within the hypothalamic-pituitary-adrenocortical axis
            (2) Possible diminished release of thyroid-stimulating hormone
         d. Physiological influences
            (1) Medication side effects
            (2) Neurological disorders
            (3) Electrolyte disturbances
            (4) Hormonal disorders
            (5) Nutritional deficiencies
            (6) Other physiological conditions
      2. Psychosocial theories
         a. Psychoanalytical theories
            (1) Freud: a loss is internalized and becomes directed against the ego.
            (2) Klein: the result of a poor mother-infant relationship.
         b. Learning theory: learned helplessness. The individual who experiences numerous failures learns to give up trying.
         c. Object loss theory: occurs when an individual is separated from a significant other during the first 6 months of life.
         d. Cognitive theory: cognitive distortions result in negative, defeatist attitudes that serve as the basis for depression.
         e. Theoretical integration. Exact etiology of depression remains unclear. Evidence continues to mount in support of multiple causation.
   B. Developmental implications
      1. Childhood depression
      2. Adolescence
      3. Senescence
      4. **Postpartum depression**
   C. Application of the nursing process to depressive disorders

1. Background assessment data
   a. Symptoms occur by degree of severity and may be ranked as transient, mild, moderate, or severe.
   b. Transient: life's everyday disappointments that result in the "blues"
   c. Mild depression: identified with those symptoms of normal grieving
   d. Moderate depression: identified by those symptoms associated with dysthymic disorder
   e. Severe depression: identified by those symptoms associated with major depressive disorder and bipolar depression
2. Nursing diagnoses are formulated by analyzing the data gathered during the assessment phase of the nursing process. Outcome criteria are identified for each.
3. Client/family education
4. Nursing interventions for the depressed client are aimed at:
   a. Protecting client from harming self.
   b. Assisting with progression through the grief process.
   c. Enhancing client's self-esteem.
   d. Helping the client determine ways to take control over his or her life.
   e. Assisting client in confronting anger that has been turned inward on the self.
   f. Ensuring that needs related to nutrition, elimination, activity, rest, and personal hygiene are met.
4. Evaluation of the effectiveness of nursing interventions is measured by fulfillment of the outcome criteria.

VI. Bipolar Disorder (Mania)
   A. Etiological implications
      1. Biological theories
         a. Genetics. Strong hereditary implications
         b. Biochemical influences. Possible excess of norepinephrine and dopamine
         c. Electrolytes. Increased intracellular sodium and calcium has been implicated.
         d. Physiological influences
            (1) Brain lesions
            (2) Medication side effects
      2. Psychosocial theories: Credibility has been questioned.
      3. Mood disorders can likely be attributed to multiple causation.
   B. Application of the nursing process to bipolar disorder (mania)
      1. Background assessment data
         a. Symptoms may be categorized by degree of severity.
         b. Stage I. **Hypomania:** symptoms not sufficiently severe to cause marked impairment in social or occupational functioning or to require hospitalization
         c. Stage II. Acute mania: marked impairment in functioning of mood, cognition and perception, activity, and behavior; usually requires hospitalization

      d. Stage III. **Delirious mania:** a grave form of the disorder characterized by severe clouding of consciousness and representing an intensification of the symptoms associated with acute mania

  2. Nursing diagnoses are formulated by analyzing the data gathered during the assessment phase of the nursing process. Outcome criteria are identified for each.

  3. Client/family education

  4. Nursing interventions for the client experiencing a manic episode are aimed at:
      a. Protection from injury due to hyperactivity.
      b. Protection from harm to self or others.
      c. Restoration of nutritional status.
      d. Progression toward resolution of the grief process.
      e. Improvement in interactions with others.
      f. Acquiring sufficient rest and sleep.

  5. Evaluation of the effectiveness of the nursing interventions is measured by fulfillment of the outcome criteria.

VII. Treatment Modalities for Mood Disorders
  A. Psychological treatments
    1. Individual psychotherapy
    2. Group therapy
    3. Family therapy
    4. **Cognitive therapy**
  B. Organic treatments
    1. Psychopharmacology
    2. **Electroconvulsive therapy**

VIII. Suicide
  A. Epidemiological factors
  B. Facts and fables about suicide
  C. Risk factors associated with suicide
  D. Nursing care of the suicidal client

IX. Summary

X. Critical Thinking Exercise

XI. Review Questions

ANSWERS TO CRITICAL THINKING EXERCISE

1. Protection from injury and adequate nutrition and rest
2. Evidence of full manic episode
3. Ataxia, blurred vision, persistent diarrhea, nausea and vomiting, tinnitis
4. Lithium does not take effect for 1 to 3 weeks. Thorazine was ordered to calm her hyperactivity until the lithium takes effect.

CASE STUDIES FOR USE WITH STUDENT LEARNING

Case Study No. 1: Major Depressive Disorder

Valerie, age 25, is admitted to the psychiatric unit by her psychiatrist after stating that she no longer wanted to live. She has a long history of psychiatric problems, beginning at age 15, when she swallowed a handful of aspirin and acetaminophen. Valerie's mother has a history of depression and her father is very authoritarian. He ruled Valerie and her sister with an iron hand, and rarely showed affection or gave positive feedback. In college Valerie met Bob, with whom she immediately fell in love. He was very affectionate, and she felt she received some nurturing from him that she had not received from her parents. In the semester before graduation, Bob told her he was leaving to go to graduate school in another state, and that he was not ready to get married at this time. Valerie became hysterical and went into a deep depression. After a few weeks she met Jack, with whom she immediately began a sexual relationship and became pregnant. Jack agreed to marry Valerie, and so they began a short, but extremely stormy, relationship. Six months after the birth of their baby boy, they began divorce proceedings with a great deal of negative negotiations regarding custody and child support. The child is 4 years old now, and Valerie has had several "serious" relationships since her divorce, having just broken off from the most recent one this week. Ralph told her that she is just "too intense, draining him of all his energy." She said he told her that she expects too much from their relationship—more than he has to give. She admits that she got serious really fast, but that she really believes she loves him. She says to the admitting nurse, "What's the matter with me? Why can't I have normal relationships like other people? If it weren't for my little boy, I wouldn't even be here now." Design a plan of care for Valerie's hospital stay.

Case Study No. 2: Bipolar Mania

Noreen, age 32, had always been described as "moody." Depending upon what was happening in her life at the time, she could be very sad and depressed, or very lighthearted and happy. During her "down" times she would feel tired, experience loss of appetite, and sleep a lot. During her "happy" times, she would party a lot, be very outgoing, and have a remarkable amount of energy. Noreen did well in college and graduated at age 26 with an MBA. Since that time, she has been employed in the administration department of a large corporation, in which she has had several promotions. Two weeks ago, management was to make the announcement of who would be fulfilling the position of Vice President of Corporate Affairs. Noreen and a male colleague, Ted, were vying for the position. It was a choice position that Noreen desperately wanted. She became very depressed when the announcement was made that Ted had been chosen. She stayed at home in bed and slept a lot for several days. On about the 4th day, she got up, feeling exhilarated, and decided to go shopping. She spent over a thousand dollars on clothing. She then decided to have a party for several hundred people, ordered catering, and planned all the details. Tonight was the party. Noreen wore a new, very expensive dress, drank a lot of champagne, was very jovial and seductive, and bragged to everyone who would listen that she would soon be getting a new job, and that the people at her old organization would be sorry they had failed to promote her. She left the party with a man she hardly knew. At 3:00 A.M., she was picked up by the police, under the grandstand at the local baseball stadium, wearing only her underclothes and high heeled shoes, and carrying a half-filled bottle of champagne. She was alone, and speaking very loudly and rapidly. The police brought her to the emergency department where she was admitted to the psychiatric unit with a diagnosis of Manic Episode. Design an initial care plan for Noreen.

LEARNING ACTIVITY

Symptoms of Mood Disorders

Beside each of the behaviors listed below, write the letter that identifies the disorder in which the behavior is most prevalent. The first one is completed as an example.

a. Dysthymic Disorder	d. Cyclothymic Disorder
b. Major Depressive Disorder	e. Bipolar Disorder (Mania)

c. Transient Depression   f. Delirious Mania

__c__ 1. Feeling of the "blues" in response to everyday disappointments.

_____ 2. A clouding of consciousness occurs.

_____ 3. Outlook is gloomy and pessimistic.

_____ 4. Characterized by mood swings between hypomania and mild depression.

_____ 5. Feelings of total despair and hopelessness.

_____ 6. Physical movement may come to a standstill.

_____ 7. Paranoid and grandiose delusions are common.

_____ 8. Feels at their best early in the morning and continually feels worse as the day progresses.

_____ 9. Excessive interest in sexual activity.

_____ 10. Able to carry out thoughts of self-destructive behavior.

_____ 11. Feels at their worst early in the morning and somewhat better as the day progresses.

_____ 12. Accelerated, pressured speech.

_____ 13. Frenzied motor activity characterized by agitated, purposeless movements.

TEST QUESTIONS

Situation: Janet, age 28, was diagnosed at age 24 with Bipolar Disorder. The physician prescribed lithium carbonate 300 mg t.i.d. for maintenance therapy. Janet lives at home with her parents. Her mother reports that Janet quit taking her lithium about 3 months ago, stating that she felt just fine and didn't like taking the medication because it was making her gain weight. Her behavior has become more and more hyperactive. She has slept very little. She has managed to maintain her office job, but today Janet's mother got a call from Janet's boss saying that Janet had lost her temper, started yelling and cursing at the other people in the office, and walked out yelling that she didn't need this job anymore. The police were called by a downtown department store when Janet became aggressive and belligerent after being confronted for shoplifting. She was taken to the emergency department of the local hospital, and her parents were notified that she had been admitted to the psychiatric unit.

1. Janet is agitated, pacing, talking loudly and abusively as if in response to an unseen person, and flailing her arms in exaggerated gestures. She is begun on lithium carbonate and haloperidol (Haldol) immediately. What is the rationale for the haloperidol order?

a. Haloperidol cures manic symptoms.
b. Haloperidol prevents extrapyramidal side effects.
c. Haloperidol will ensure that she gets a good night's sleep.
- d. Haloperidol will calm hyperactivity until lithium takes effect.

2. At this level of her illness, the nurse caring for Janet must consider which of the following nursing diagnoses as the priority?
   - a. Risk for injury related to excessive hyperactivity
   b. Sleep pattern disturbance related to manic hyperactivity
   c. Alteration in nutrition, less than body requirements related to inadequate intake
   d. Self-esteem disturbance related to embarrassment from being arrested for shoplifting

3. Janet tells the physician that she does not want to take lithium carbonate because she has gained a lot of weight on this medication. She says that if he sends her home on this drug, she will just stop taking it again. The physician decides to change her medication in hopes that she will be more compliant. Which of the following medications might the physician choose to prescribe for Janet?
   a. sertraline (Zoloft)
   - b. valproic acid (Depakote)
   c. trazodone (Desyrel)
   d. paroxetine (Paxil)

Janet is stabilized on her medication and the hyperactivity subsides. She is discharged from the hospital to her parent's home. She apologizes to her boss for her behavior and is rehired. Because of cutbacks and downsizing 10 months later, however, Janet is laid off. She becomes very depressed, refuses to look for another job, stays in her room, eats very little, and neglects her personal hygiene. She tells her mother, "What's the use of trying? I fail at everything I do, anyway. Nothing ever works out for me." The next morning, when Janet's mother goes in to check on her, she finds Janet unconscious but still breathing, with an empty bottle of sertraline (Zoloft) beside her. She calls an ambulance and has Janet transported to the hospital emergency department. Janet is stabilized in the ED and admitted to the psychiatric unit. Her diagnosis is Bipolar I Disorder: Current Episode Depressed.

4. Why does the physician give Janet this diagnosis rather than major depression?
   a. Because he doesn't feel she is that severely depressed.
   - b. Because she has experienced a full manic episode in the past.
   c. Because he needs to make a more extensive assessment before he decides.
   d. Because she has no history of major depression in her family.

5. What would be the *priority* nursing diagnosis for Janet at this time?
   a. Alteration in nutrition, less than body requirements, related to refusal to eat
   b. Anxiety (severe) related to threat to self-esteem
   - c. Risk for suicide related to depressed mood
   d. Dysfunctional grieving related to loss of employment

6. The physician prescribes paroxetine (Paxil) for Janet. She is encouraged to participate in unit activities and to talk about her feelings. Despite all efforts, her depression becomes profound. She is in total despair and in a vegetative state. The physician obtains consent from her parents to perform ECT. What is the rationale behind this treatment for profound depression?
   a. The client is made to forget painful memories from the past and go on with his or her life.
   b. The treatment causes stimulation of the central nervous system similar to CNS stimulant medication, thereby lifting mood.
   c. The treatment satisfies the need for punishment that severely depressed clients sometimes think they deserve.
   - d. The treatment is thought to increase levels of norepinephrine and serotonin, resulting in mood elevation.

7. The physician orders a medication to be administered by the nurse 30 minutes prior to each ECT treatment that will decrease secretions and maintain heart rate during the convulsion. Which of the following medications would the physician prescribe for this purpose?
   a. Thiopental sodium (Pentothal)
   - b. Atropine sulfate
   c. Succinylcholine (Anectine)
   d. Clonazepam (Klonopin)

8. Which of the following currently receives the most credibility as etiologically implicated in the development of bipolar disorder?
   - a. Genetics and biochemical alterations
   b. Poor mother-child relationship
   c. Evidence of lesion in temporal lobe
   d. Learned helplessness within a dysfunctional family system

9. Which of the following individuals is considered at highest risk for suicide?
   a. 45-year-old African American female
   b. 50-year-old married, Jewish farmer
   - c. 65-year-old widowed, protestant lawyer

d. 25-year-old Hispanic female, married and Catholic

10. A client who is prescribed an MAO inhibitor for depression should have which of the following as part of his or her medication education?
    a. There is a possibility of sexual dysfunction with this medication.
    b. Maintain adequate protection from the sun because of the side effect of photosensitivity.
    c. This medication may cause pulse irregularities.
    • d. Don't eat foods containing tyramine while taking this medication.

CHAPTER 16. ANXIETY DISORDERS

CHAPTER FOCUS

The focus of this chapter is on nursing care of the client with anxiety disorders. Etiological implications and symptomatology are explored, and nursing care is presented in the context of the six steps of the nursing process. Medical treatment modalities are also discussed.

LEARNING OBJECTIVES

After reading this chapter, the student will be able to:
1. Differentiate among the terms *stress*, *anxiety*, and *fear*.
2. Discuss historical aspects and epidemiological statistics related to anxiety disorders.
3. Differentiate between normal anxiety and psychoneurotic anxiety.
4. Describe various types of anxiety disorders and identify symptomatology associated with each. Use this information in client assessment.
5. Identify etiological implications in the development of anxiety disorders.
6. Formulate nursing diagnoses and outcome criteria for clients with anxiety disorders.
7. Describe appropriate nursing interventions for behaviors associated with anxiety disorders.
8. Evaluate nursing care of clients with anxiety disorders.
9. Discuss various modalities relevant to treatment of anxiety disorders.

KEY TERMS

agoraphobia
flooding
generalized anxiety disorder
implosion therapy
obsessive-compulsive disorder
panic disorder
phobias
posttraumatic stress disorder
ritualistic behavior
specific phobia
social phobia
systematic desensitization

CHAPTER OUTLINE/LECTURE NOTES

I. Introduction
   A. Anxiety is a necessary force for survival. It is not the same as stress.

B. Stress (or stressor) is an external pressure that is brought to bear on the individual. Anxiety is the subjective emotional response to that stressor.

C. Anxiety is distinguished from fear in that anxiety is an emotional process whereas fear is a cognitive one.

II. Historical Aspects

A. Anxiety was once identified by its physiological symptoms, focusing largely on the cardiovascular system.

B. Freud was the first to associate anxiety with neurotic behaviors.

C. For many years, anxiety disorders were viewed as purely psychological or purely biological in nature.

III. Epidemiological Statistics

A. Anxiety disorders represent one of the most prevalent mental health problems in the United States today.

B. Anxiety disorders are more common in women than in men.

IV. How Much is Too Much?

A. Anxiety is pathological if:

1. The response is greatly disproportionate to the risk and severity of the danger or threat.

2. The response continues beyond the existence of a potential danger or threat.

3. Intellectual, social, or occupational functioning is impaired.

4. The individual suffers from a psychosomatic effect (for example, colitis or dermatitis).

V. Application of the Nursing Process

A. Panic disorder

1. Background assessment data

a. Characterized by recurrent panic attacks, the onset of which are unpredictable and manifested by intense apprehension, fear, or terror, often associated with feelings of impending doom, and accompanied by intense physical discomfort

(1) Palpitations, pounding heart, or accelerated heart rate

(2) Sweating

(3) Trembling or shaking

(4) Sensations of shortness of breath or smothering

(5) Feeling of choking

(6) Chest pain or discomfort

(7) Nausea or abdominal distress

(8) Feeling dizzy, unsteady, lightheaded, or faint

(9) Derealization (feelings of unreality) or depersonalization (being detached from oneself)

(10) Fear of losing control or going crazy

(11) Fear of dying

(12) Parethesias (numbness or tingling sensations)

(13) Chills or hot flashes

b. With **agoraphobia**: When panic disorder is accompanied by agoraphobia, the individual experiences the symptoms described above, but in addition, experiences a fear of being in places or situations from which escape might be difficult or embarrassing or in which help might not be available in the event of a panic attack.

B. **Generalized anxiety disorder**
 1. Background assessment data
   a. Characterized by chronic, unrealistic, and excessive anxiety and worry Symptoms include:
    (1) Excessive anxiety and worry about a number of events that the individual finds difficult to control.
    (2) Restlessness or feeling keyed up or on edge.
    (3) Being easily fatigued.
    (4) Difficulty concentrating or mind "going blank."
    (5) Irritability.
    (6) Muscle tension.
    (7) Sleep disturbance.
 2. Etiological implications for panic and generalized anxiety disorders
   a. Psychodynamic theory. An underdeveloped ego is not able to intervene when conflict occurs between the id and the superego, producing anxiety.
   b. Cognitive theory. This theory places emphasis on distorted cognition, which results in anxiety that is maintained by mistaken or dysfunctional appraisal of a situation.
   c. Biological aspects
    (1) Neuroanatomical. The lower brain centers may be responsible for initiating and controlling states of physiological arousal and for the involuntary homeostatic functions.
    (2) Biochemical. Abnormal elevations of blood lactate have been noted in clients with panic disorder.
    (3) Neurochemical. Evidence exists for the involvement of the neurotransmitter norepinephrine in the etiology of panic disorder.
    (4) Medical conditions. Various medical conditions, such as acute MI, hypoglycemia, mitral valve prolapse, and complex partial seizures, have been associated to a greater degree with individuals who suffer from panic and generalized anxiety disorders than in the general population.
 3. Diagnosis/outcome identification
   a. Nursing diagnoses are formulated from the data gathered during the assessment phase.
    (1) Panic anxiety
    (2) Powerlessness
   b. Outcome criteria are used as measurement guidelines to evaluate effectiveness of nursing care.
 4. Planning/implementation
   a. Nursing intervention for the client with panic or generalized anxiety disorder is aimed at relief of acute panic symptoms.

    b. The nurse also works at assisting the client to take control of own life situation and accept those situations over which he or she has no control.
  5. Evaluation is based on accomplishment of previously established outcome criteria.

C. **Phobias**
  1. Background assessment data
    a. Agoraphobia without history of panic disorder. A fear of being in places or situations from which escape might be difficult, or in which help might not be available in the event of suddenly developing a panic or limited symptom attack.
    b. **Social phobia.** Characterized by an excessive fear of situations in which a person might do something embarrassing or be evaluated negatively by others.
    c. **Specific phobia.** A marked, persistent, and excessive or unreasonable fear when in the presence of, or when anticipating an encounter with, a specific object or situation.
  2. Etiological implications for phobias
    a. Psychoanalytical theory. Freud believed that during the Oedipal period, the child becomes frightened of the aggression he fears that the same sex parents feels for him. This fear is repressed and displaced onto something safer, which becomes the phobic stimulus.
    b. Learning theory. Learning theorists believe that fears are learned and become conditioned responses when the individual escapes panic anxiety (a negative reinforcement) by avoiding the phobic stimulus.
    c. Cognitive theory. Cognitive theorists espouse that anxiety is the product of faulty cognitions or anxiety-inducing self-instructions.
    d. Biological aspects
      (1) Temperament. Innate fears may represent a part of the overall characteristics or tendencies with which one is born that influence how one responds throughout life to specific situations.
      (2) Life experiences. Certain early experiences may set the stage for phobic reactions later in life.
  3. Diagnosis/outcome identification
    a. Nursing diagnoses are formulated using information gathered during the assessment phase:
      (1) Fear
      (2) Social isolation
    b. Outcome criteria are used as measurement guidelines to evaluate effectiveness of nursing care.
  4. Planning/implementation. Nursing intervention for the client with phobias is aimed at decreasing the fear and increasing the ability to function in the presence of the phobic stimulus.
  5. Evaluation is based on accomplishment of previously established outcome criteria.

D. **Obsessive-compulsive disorder**

1. Background assessment data. Recurrent obsessions or compulsions that are severe enough to be time consuming or to cause marked distress or significant impairment.
2. Etiological implications for obsessive-compulsive disorder
   a. Psychoanalytical theory. Individuals with this disorder have weak, underdeveloped egos. Regression to the pre-Oedipal phase of development during times of anxiety produce the symptoms of obsessions and compulsions.
   b. Learning theory. Obsessive-compulsive behavior is viewed as a conditioned response to a traumatic event. The traumatic event produces anxiety and discomfort, and the individual learns to prevent it by avoiding the situation with which it is associated.
   c. Biological aspects
      (1) Neuroanatomy. Abnormalities in various regions of the brain have been implicated in the neurobiology of obsessive-compulsive disorder.
      (2) Physiology. Some individuals with obsessive-compulsive disorder exhibit nonspecific EEG changes.
      (3) Biochemical. A decrease in the neurotransmitter serotonin may be influential in the etiology of obsessive-compulsive disorder.
3. Diagnosis/outcome identification
   a. Nursing diagnoses are formulated from the assessment data gathered during the first phase:
      (1) Ineffective individual coping
      (2) Altered role performance
   b. Outcome criteria are used as measurement guidelines to evaluate effectiveness of nursing care.
4. Planning/implementation. Nursing intervention of the client with obsessive-compulsive disorder is aimed at helping him or her maintain anxiety at a manageable level without having to resort to use of **ritualistic behavior**. The focus is on development of more adaptive methods of coping with anxiety.
5. Evaluation is based on accomplishment of previously established outcome criteria.
E. **Posttraumatic stress disorder** (PTSD)
   1. Background assessment data
      a. The development of characteristic symptoms following exposure to an extreme traumatic stressor involving a personal threat to physical integrity or to the physical integrity of others
      b. Symptoms may include a re-experiencing of the traumatic event, a sustained high level of anxiety or arousal, or general numbing of responsiveness.
   2. Etiological implications for PTSD
      a. Psychosocial theory
         (1) Seeks to explain why some individuals exposed to massive trauma develop PTSD whereas others do not.

    (2) Variables include characteristics that relate to the traumatic experience, the individual, and the recovery environment.

   b. Learning theory. The avoidance behaviors and psychic numbing in response to a trauma are mediated by negative reinforcement (behaviors that decrease the emotional pain of the trauma).

   c. Cognitive theory. Takes into consideration the cognitive appraisal of an event and focuses on assumptions that an individual makes about the world.

   d. Biological aspects. It is suggested that the symptoms related to the trauma are maintained by the production of endogenous opioid peptides that are produced in the face of arousal, and that result in increased feelings of comfort and control. When the stressor terminates, the individual may experience opioid withdrawal, the symptoms of which bear strong resemblance to those of PTSD.

  3. Diagnosis/outcome identification

   a. Nursing diagnoses are formulated from the data collected during the assessment phase:

    (1) Posttrauma response

    (2) Dysfunctional grieving

   b. Outcome criteria are used as measurement guidelines to evaluate effectiveness of nursing care.

  4. Planning/implementation

   a. Nursing intervention for the client with PTSD is aimed at:

    (1) Reassurance of safety.

    (2) Decrease in maladaptive symptoms (for example, flashbacks, nightmares).

    (3) Demonstration of more adaptive coping strategies.

    (4) Adaptive progression through the grief process.

  5. Evaluation is based on accomplishment of previously established outcome criteria.

 F. Anxiety disorder due to a general medical condition

  1. Background assessment data

   a. The symptoms are judged to be the direct physiological consequence of a general medical condition.

   b. Symptoms may include generalized anxiety symptoms, panic attacks, or obsessions and compulsions.

 G. Substance-induced anxiety disorder

  1. Background assessment data

   a. Prominent anxiety symptoms that are judged to be due to the direct physiological effects of a substance.

   b. Symptoms may occur during substance intoxication or withdrawal, and may involve prominent anxiety, panic attacks, phobias, or obsessions or compulsions.

 H. Topics for client/family education related to anxiety disorders

VI. Treatment Modalities for Anxiety Disorders

A. Individual psychotherapy
B. Cognitive therapy
C. Behavior therapy
   1. **Systematic desensitization**
   2. **Implosion therapy (flooding)**
D. Group/family therapy
E. Psychopharmacology

VII. Summary

VIII. Critical Thinking Exercise

XI. Review Questions

ANSWERS TO CRITICAL THINKING EXERCISE

1. Panic anxiety related to threat to self-concept (fear of failure)

2. Stay with her and reassure her of her safety.

3. A benzodiazepine (for example, clonazepam, alprazolam, or lorazepam) and individual psychotherapy

CASE STUDIES FOR USE WITH STUDENT LEARNING

Case Study No. 1: Obsessive-Compulsive Disorder

Lana, age 28, has been admitted to the psychiatric unit with a diagnosis of OCD. She has been under the care of a psychiatrist since she was 14 years old. At that time she was diagnosed with Anorexia Nervosa. She was treated for that disease, stabilized, and her family underwent counseling for about 1 year. She had a mild recurrence of the disease during her college years, but was treated on an outpatient basis. Lana reported to the admitting nurse that during the last few years she has become increasingly obsessed with neatness and cleanliness. She washes her hands many times a day, and when possible, changes her clothing several times a day. She spends an enormous amount of time doing laundry and cleaning her apartment. Her hands crack and bleed from the excessive hand washing. She takes hours to get ready to go somewhere. If the routine is interrupted in any way, she starts over from the beginning. Recently she got up at 1:30 A.M. to start getting ready for work. She has also started to lose weight again. She has a poor body image, and although her weight is appropriate for her height, she sees herself as overweight. She tells the nurse that she knows her behavior is inappropriate, but she can't seem to stop herself. Design a care plan for Lana.

Case Study No. 2: Posttraumatic Stress Disorder

Sarah, age 25, graduated from college with a degree in journalism. She was thrilled to obtain a position as a reporter with a local TV station. She has been working as a production assistant for 6 months, and was recently promoted to reporter. About a month ago, she received the police alert of someone about to jump off a tall building, and was dispatched with a photographer to the scene. For several hours, she witnessed the scene unravel as the police tried in vain to keep the man from jumping. Sarah watched with horror as the man jumped 20 stories to his death. She had always believed that she could be objective about such events and not have them affect her personally, but since that time she has thought about the event on a daily basis. She has flashbacks and nightmares of seeing the man fall, and lately she has been reluctant even to go to work. Her boss suggests that she seek the assistance of a psychiatrist. She is admitted to the partial hospitalization program with a diagnosis of PTSD. Design a nursing plan of care for Sarah during her partial hospitalization.

LEARNING ACTIVITY

BEHAVIORS ASSOCIATED WITH ANXIETY DISORDERS

Identify with which anxiety disorder the behaviors listed are associated. The first one is completed as an example.

a. Panic disorder
b. Agoraphobia
c. Posttraumatic stress disorder

e. Generalized anxiety disorder
f. Social phobia
g. Obsessive-compulsive disorder

__c__ 1. Janet becomes panicky when she gets near a dog.

_____ 2. Patricia weighs and measures her food. Long after everyone else has finished eating, she is still calculating the caloric value and remeasuring the amount.

_____ 3. Frances will not leave her home unless a friend or relative goes with her.

_____ 4. Harold has intrusive thoughts and sometimes visual illusions of his platoon's invasion of a village in Vietnam.

_____ 5. Sonja refuses to eat in a restaurant. She is afraid others will laugh at the way she eats.

_____ 6. About once a week, without warning, Stanley's heart begins to pound, he becomes short of breath, and sometimes he experiences chest pain. The doctor has ruled out physical problems.

_____ 7. Janie wants desperately to visit a foreign country with her friends, but because of her fear of needles, she has not been able to receive the required immunizations.

_____ 8. Helen is a very restless person. She is always nervous and keyed up. She worries about many things over which she has no control.

_____ 9. Timmie's family recently survived a tornado by taking refuge in the basement of their home. The home and all of its contents were destroyed. Timmie has nightmares about the event.

_____ 10. George never volunteers to speak in class. He is afraid his classmates will laugh at what he says.

_____ 11. Carl will go to church, but only if he can sit right near the door.

_____ 12. When Sally sees a spider on the floor, she screams and runs out of the room.

_____ 13. Every day when Wanda goes home from work, she cleans her house. She has told her friends not to call her during this time, and if anything interferes with her cleaning, she becomes very upset, and starts over from the beginning.

_____ 14. Don has always been an excellent student and was valedictorian of his high school graduating class. Since starting college, he has been unusually worried about his academic performance. Lately, he has been unable to sleep, is irritable, has difficulty concentrating, and has begun experiencing nausea and vomiting because he is worried that he will not do well academically.

_____ 15. Last month, on her way out of the hospital after working the evening shift, Amanda was abducted by a man with a gun and taken to a remote area and raped. Since that time, she has become detached and estranged from her friends, she has difficulty sleeping, and has had problems concentrating at work.

TEST QUESTIONS

Situation: Sharon is a 25-year-old graduate student working on a doctorate in pharmacy. She is very bright and very achievement oriented. She works very hard and pushes herself to excel. Lately, she has been very upset because she isn't studying as much as she usually does, and she is afraid she will fail some of her courses. She has begun cleaning out her drawers and closets incessantly. If she notices one thing out of place, she removes the entire contents and begins to rearrange them. Many times during the ritual, she gets interrupted and starts all over again. She knows that the behavior is not normal, but she feels powerless to change. She has been admitted to the psychiatric unit with the diagnosis of obsessive-compulsive disorder.

1. After her initial assessment and introduction to the unit, Sharon goes to her room to unpack her suitcase. She begins to arrange her belongings in the drawers and closet. Forty-five minutes later, when the nurse comes to check on her, Sharon is still folding and unfolding her clothes, and arranging and rearranging them in the drawers. What is the appropriate nursing intervention at this time?
    a. Explain to Sharon that she must come out of her room and join the others in the dayroom at this time.
    b. Give Sharon a task to complete, to get her mind off the ritual.
  • c. Allow Sharon as much time as she wants to perform the ritual.
    d. Take Sharon by the hand and state, "It's time to go to group therapy now."

2. The most likely reason Sharon arranges and rearranges her clothing so often is:
  • a. It relieves her anxiety.
    b. Her mother taught her to be very neat.
    c. It provides her with a feeling of control over her life.
    d. It makes her feel good about herself.

3. The physician writes an order for medication for Sharon. Which of the following is an appropriate prescription for obsessive-compulsive disorder?
    a. Diazepam (Valium)
  • b. Fluvoxamine (Luvox)
    c. Propranolol (Inderal)
    d. Alprazolam (Xanax)

4. Which of the following would be an appropriate nursing intervention with Sharon?

a. Distract Sharon with other activities whenever she tries to clean out her drawers.

b. Report the behavior to the physician each time she begins the ritual.

c. Lock Sharon's room so that she cannot engage in the ritualistic behavior.

- d. Help Sharon identify what is causing the anxiety that leads to the ritualistic behavior.

5. As Sharon becomes more comfortable on the unit, and begins to interact with others, what change, if any, should the nurse make in her plan of care?
    - a. Begin to set limits on the amount of time Sharon may engage in the ritual.
    b. Give negative reinforcement to the behavior by pointing out its inappropriateness.
    c. Establish firm consequences if Sharon performs the ritualistic behavior.
    d. No change should be made in the plan of care.

6. Recently, the biochemical theory of etiology of obsessive-compulsive disorder has been given an increasing amount of credibility. Which neurotransmitter has been associated with this disorder?
    a. Norepinephrine
    b. Dopamine
    - c. Serotonin
    d. Acetylcholine

7. Which of the following medications might you expect a physician to prescribe for a client with posttraumatic stress disorder who is experiencing intrusive recollections, flashbacks, and nightmares?
    a. Clomipramine (Anafranil)
    b. Clozapine (Clozaril)
    c. Diazepam (Valium)
    - d. Carbamazepine (Tegretol)

8. Sally is diagnosed with panic disorder. She experiences symptoms such as palpitations, trembling, sensation of shortness of breath, chest pain, and chills or hot flashes. An appropriate outcome in working with Sally is for her to be able to:
    a. Monitor her own blood pressure.
    - b. Interrupt progression of escalating anxiety.
    c. Premedicate herself to prevent panic symptoms.
    d. Identify support sources to call upon in the event of a panic attack.

9. The psychiatrist asks his nurse to interview Mrs. Smith, who has been diagnosed with acrophobia. The nurse would expect Mrs. Smith to have an intense fear of:
   - • a. Traveling by airplane
     b. Spiders
     c. Riding in a car
     d. 13 persons at a table

10. When a client is experiencing panic anxiety, the priority nursing intervention is:
    a. Helping the client recognize what brought on the attack.
    b. Use reality orientation to show the client that he or she need not be afraid.
    - • c. Reassuring the client that he or she is safe.
    d. Encouraging the client to explore underlying feelings that may be contributing to irrational fears.

CHAPTER 17. ANXIETY-RELATED DISORDERS

CHAPTER FOCUS

The focus of this chapter is on nursing care of individuals experiencing various disorders associated with anxiety. Etiological implications and symptomatology are explored, and nursing care is presented in the context of the six steps of the nursing process. Medical treatment modalities are also discussed.

LEARNING OBJECTIVES

After reading this chapter, the student will be able to:
1. Discuss historical aspects and epidemiological statistics related to psychophysiological, somatoform, and dissociative disorders.
2. Describe various types of psychophysiological, somatoform, and dissociative disorders and identify symptomatology associated with each; use this information in client assessment.
3. Identify etiological implications in the development of psychophysiological, somatoform, and dissociative disorders.
4. Formulate nursing diagnoses and goals of care for clients with psychophysiological, somatoform, and dissociative disorders.
5. Describe appropriate nursing interventions for behaviors associated with psychophysiological, somatoform, and dissociative disorders.
6. Evaluate the nursing care of clients with psychophysiological, somatoform, and dissociative disorders.
7. Discuss various modalities relevant to treatment of psychophysiological, somatoform, and dissociative disorders.

KEY TERMS

Autoimmune	carcinogens
psychophysiological	type A personality
type B personality	type C personality
abreaction	amnesia
derealization	depersonalization
fugue	integration
anosmia	aphonia
hypochondriasis	hysteria
primary gain	la belle indifference
secondary gain	pseudocyesis
tertiary gain	somatization

CHAPTER OUTLINE/LECTURE NOTES
I. Introduction

A. **Psychophysiological** responses to anxiety are those in which it has been determined that psychological factors contribute to the initiation or exacerbation of the physical condition. Evidence *does* exist to support the presence of organic pathology or a known pathophysiological process.

B. Somatoform disorders are characterized by physical symptoms suggesting medical disease, but without a demonstrable organic pathology or known pathophysiological mechanism to account for them.

C. Dissociative disorders are defined by a disruption in the usually integrated functions of consciousness, memory, identity, or perception of the environment.

II. Historical Aspects

   A. For more than a century, physicians have agreed that in some disorders there is an interaction between emotional and physical factors.

   B. Historically, somatoform disorders have been identified as *hysterical neuroses*. Somatoform disorders are thought to occur in response to repressed severe anxiety.

   C. Freud viewed dissociation as a type of repression, an active defense mechanism used to remove threatening or unacceptable mental contents from conscious awareness.

III. Epidemiological Statistics

   A. Somatoform disorders are more common in women than in men. They are more common in those who are poorly educated, live in rural communities, and are in the lower socioeconomic classes.

   B. Dissociative disorders are thought to be quite rare, with **amnesia** being the most common dissociative symptom. Dissociative identity disorder (DID) is more common in women than it is in men. Brief episodes of **depersonalization** symptoms appear to be common in young adulthood, particularly in times of severe stress.

IV. Application of the Nursing Process

   A. Background assessment data: Types of psychophysiological disorders

      1. Asthma

         a. A syndrome of airflow limitation characterized by increased responsiveness of the tracheobronchial tree to various stimuli and manifested by airway smooth muscle contraction, hypersecretion of mucus, and inflammation

         b. Affects approximately 10 million adults and children in the U.S.

         c. Etiological influences

            (1) Hereditary factors

            (2) Allergies

            (3) Psychosocial influences: excessive dependence needs

         d. Medical treatment modalities

            (1) Pharmacotherapy

            (2) Individual psychotherapy

      2. Cancer

         a. A malignant neoplasm in which the basic structure and activity of the cells have become deranged, usually because of changes in the DNA.

b. Cancer is the second leading cause of death in the United States today.
c. Etiological influences
    (1) Hereditary factors
    (2) Environmental factors
    (3) Psychosocial influences: type C personality
d. Medical treatment modalities
    (1) Surgery
    (2) Radiation therapy
    (3) Chemotherapy
    (4) Individual psychotherapy
3. Coronary heart disease
    a. Myocardial impairment caused by an imbalance between coronary blood flow and myocardial oxygen requirements caused by changes in the coronary circulation.
    b. It is the leading cause of death in the United States
    c. Etiological influences
        (1) Hereditary factors
        (2) Environmental factors
        (3) Psychosocial influences: **Type A personality**
    d. Medical treatment modalities
        (1) Pharmacotherapy
        (2) Behavior modification
4. Peptic ulcer
    a. An erosion of the mucosal wall in the esophagus, stomach, duodenum, or jejunum
    b. More common in men than in women. Affects up to 10 percent of the general population
    c. Etiological influences
        (1) Hereditary factors
        (2) Environmental factors
        (3) Psychosocial influences: unfulfilled dependency needs
    d. Medical treatment modalities
        (1) Pharmacotherapy
        (2) Dietary intervention
        (3) Individual psychotherapy
5. Essential hypertension
    a. The persistent elevation of blood pressure for which there is no apparent cause or associated underlying disease. It is the major cause of cerebrovascular accident, cardiac disease, and renal failure.
    b. Twenty-five percent of the adult population in the United States are hypertensive (blood pressure $\geq$ 140/90). Half of the people with hypertension do not know they have it. The disorder is more common in men than in women and is twice as prevalent in the black population as it is in the white population.
    c. Etiological influences

      (1) Hereditary factors

      (2) Physiological influences

      (3) Environmental factors

      (4) Psychosocial influences: repressed anger

   d. Medical treatment modalities

      (1) Lifestyle changes

      (2) Pharmacotherapy

      (3) Relaxation therapy

6. Migraine headache

   a. A vascular event in which pain arises from the scalp, its blood vessels, and muscles; from the dura mater and its venous sinuses; and from the blood vessels at the base of the brain.

   b. Approximately 5 percent of the population suffers from migraine headaches. They are more common in women than they are in men.

   c. Etiological influences

      (1) Hereditary factors

      (2) Environmental factors

      (3) Psychosocial influences: the migraine personality

   d. Medical treatment modalities

      (1) Pharmacotherapy

      (2) Relaxation therapy

      (3) Behavior modification

      (4) Dietary restrictions

      (5) Individual psychotherapy

7. Rheumatoid arthritis

   a. A disease characterized by chronic musculoskeletal pain caused by inflammatory disease of the joints. It is a systemic disease and may also be manifested by lesions of the major organs of the body.

   b. Rheumatoid arthritis is more prevalent in women than in men and affects 1 to 3 percent of the population in the United States.

   c. Etiological influences

      (1) Hereditary factors

      (2) Psychosocial influences: suppression of anger and hostility

   d. Medical treatment modalities

      (1) Pharmacological treatment

      (2) Surgical treatment

      (3) Psychotherapy

8. Ulcerative colitis

   a. A chronic inflammatory ulcerative disease of the colon.

   b. Incidence of the disease in the United States is approximately 5 to 7 per 100,000 population.

   c. Etiological influences

      (1) Hereditary factors

      (2) Psychosocial influences

         (a) Obsessive-compulsive personality

          (b) Suppression of anger and hostility
     d. Medical treatment modalities
        (1) Nutritional therapy
        (2) Pharmacological treatment
        (3) Surgical treatment
        (4) Psychological support
  B. Diagnosis/outcome identification
     1. Nursing diagnoses for clients with psychophysiological disorders may relate to symptoms of the specific disorder. Nursing diagnoses common to the general category include:
       a. Ineffective individual coping.
       b. Knowledge deficit.
       c. Self-esteem disturbance.
       d. Altered role performance.
     2. Outcome criteria are identified for measuring the effectiveness of nursing care.
  C. Planning/implementation
     1. Nursing intervention for the client with psychophysiological disorders is determined by the type of disorder with which the client presents.
     2. Emphasis is also given to helping the individual understand the correlation between emotional problems and exacerbation of the illness. The individual receives assistance in developing more adaptive coping strategies.
  D. Client/family education
  E. Evaluation is based on accomplishment of previously established outcome criteria.
V. Application of the Nursing Process
  A. Background assessment data: types of somatoform disorders
     1. **Somatization** disorder
       a. A chronic syndrome of multiple somatic symptoms that cannot be explained medically and are associated with psychosocial distress and long-term seeking of assistance from health care professionals.
       b. The disorder is chronic and anxiety, depression, and suicide ideation are frequently manifested.
       c. Drug abuse and dependence are not uncommon complications of somatization disorder.
       d. Personality characteristics: heightened emotionality, strong dependency needs, and a preoccupation with symptoms and oneself.
     2. Pain disorder
       a. The predominant disturbance in pain disorder is severe and prolonged pain that causes clinically significant distress or impairment in social, occupational, or other areas of functioning.
       b. Even when organic pathology is detected, the pain complaint may be evidenced by the correlation of a stressful situation with the onset of symptoms.
       c. The disorder may be maintained by:

(1) **Primary gains**: the symptom enables the client to avoid some unpleasant activity.

(2) **Secondary gains**: the symptom promotes emotional support or attention for the client.

(3) **Tertiary gains**: in dysfunctional families, the physical symptom may take such a position that the real issue is disregarded and remains unresolved, even though some of the conflict is relieved.

    d. Symptoms of depression and substance abuse are common.

3. **Hypochondriasis**

    a. Unrealistic or inaccurate interpretation of physical symptoms or sensations, leading to preoccupation and fear of having a serious disease.

    b. Even in the presence of medical disease, the symptoms are grossly disproportionate to the degree of pathology.

    c. Anxiety and depression are common, and obsessive-compulsive traits frequently accompany the disorder.

4. Conversion disorder

    a. A loss of or change in body function resulting from a psychological conflict, the physical symptoms of which cannot be explained by any known medical disorder or pathophysiological mechanism.

    b. The most obvious and "classic" conversion symptoms are those that suggest neurological disease, and occur following a situation that produces extreme psychological stress for the individual.

    c. The person often expresses a relative lack of concern that is out of keeping with the severity of the impairment. This lack of concern is identified as **la belle indifference** and may be a clue to the physician that the problem is psychological rather than physical.

5. Body dysmorphic disorder

    a. Characterized by the exaggerated belief that the body is deformed or defective in some specific way.

    b. Symptoms of depression and characteristics associated with obsessive-compulsive personality are common.

B. Etiological implications for somatoform disorders

1. Genetic. There are possible hereditary factors associated with somatization disorder and hypochondriasis.

2. Biochemical. Decreased levels of serotonin and endorphins may play a role in the etiology of pain disorder.

3. Psychodynamic. This theory suggests that nurturing by the mother in the early relationship is provided only conditionally, instilling a sense of insecurity in the child. The child learns to defend against this insecurity by learning to gain affection and care through illness. Conversion disorder may represent emotions associated with a traumatic event that are too unacceptable to express and so are acceptably "converted" into physical symptoms.

4. Family dynamics. In dysfunctional families, when a child becomes ill, a shift in focus is made from the open conflict to the child's illness, leaving unresolved the underlying issues that the family is unable to confront in an

open manner. Somatization brings some stability to the family and positive reinforcement to the child.

     5. Learning theory. Somatic complaints are often reinforced when the sick person learns that he or she may avoid stressful obligations or be excused from unwanted duties (primary gains); become the prominent focus of attention because of the illness (secondary gains); or relieve conflict within the family as concern is shifted to the ill person and away from the real issue (tertiary gains).

  C. Diagnosis/outcome identification

    1. Nursing diagnoses are formulated from the data gathered during the assessment phase and with background knowledge regarding etiological implications for the illness.

    2. Some common nursing diagnoses for clients with somatoform disorders include:

      a. Ineffective individual coping

      b. Chronic pain

      c. Fear

      d. Sensory-perceptual alteration

      e. Body image disturbance

    3. Outcome criteria are identified for measuring the effectiveness of nursing care.

  D. Planning/implementation

    1. Nursing care of the individual with a somatoform disorder is aimed at relief of discomfort from the physical symptom.

    2. Assistance is provided to the client in an effort to determine strategies for coping with stress by means other than preoccupation with physical symptoms.

  E. Evaluation is based on accomplishment of previously established outcome criteria.

  F. Medical treatment modalities for somatoform disorders

    1. Individual psychotherapy

    2. Group psychotherapy

    3. Behavior therapy

    4. Psychopharmacology

VI. Application of the Nursing Process

  A. Background assessment data: types of dissociative disorders

    1. Dissociative amnesia

      a. Defined as an inability to recall important personal information that is too extensive to be explained by ordinary forgetfulness, and which is not due to the direct effects of substance use or a general medical condition. Onset usually follows severe psychosocial stress.

      b. Five types of disturbance in recall:

        (1) Localized amnesia. The inability to recall all incidents associated with the traumatic event for a specific time period following the event (usually a few hours to a few days)

(2) Selective amnesia. The inability to recall only certain incidents associated with a traumatic event for a specific time period following the event

(3) Generalized amnesia. The inability to recall anything that has happened during the individual's entire lifetime, including personal identity

(4) Continuous amnesia. The inability to recall events occurring after a specific time up to and including the present

(5) Systematized amnesia. The inability to remember events that relate to a specific category of information, such as one's family, or to one particular person or event

2. Dissociative **fugue**
   a. The characteristic feature of dissociative fugue is a sudden, unexpected travel away from home or customary workplace.
   b. An individual in a fugue state is unable to recall personal identity, and assumption of a new identity is common.

3. Dissociative identity disorder
   a. Characterized by the existence of two or more personalities within a single individual.
   b. The transition from one personality to another is usually sudden, often dramatic, and usually precipitated by stress.

4. Depersonalization disorder
   a. Characterized by a temporary change in the quality of self-awareness, which often takes the form of feelings of unreality, changes in body image, feelings of detachment from the environment, or a sense of observing oneself from outside the body.
   b. Depersonalization is defined as a disturbance in the perception of oneself.
   c. **Derealization** is described as an alteration in the perception of the external environment.
   d. Symptoms of depersonalization disorder are often accompanied by anxiety, depression, fear of going insane, obsessive thoughts, somatic complaints, and a disturbance in the subjective sense of time.

B. Etiological implications for dissociative disorders
   1. Genetics. Possible hereditary factors associated with DID.
   2. Neurobiological. It is possible that dissociative amnesia and dissociative fugue may be related to alterations in the ascending reticular activating system and thalamocortical projections. EEG abnormalities have been observed in some clients with DID.
   3. Psychodynamic theory. Freud described amnesia as the result of repression of distressing mental contents from conscious awareness. Current psychodynamic explanations of dissociation are based on Freud's concepts—that is, that behaviors such as amnesia, fugue, and depersonalization behaviors are a defense against unresolved painful issues.
   4. Psychological trauma. A growing body of evidence points to the etiology of DID as a set of traumatic experiences that overwhelms the individual's

capacity to cope by any means other than dissociation. These experiences usually take the form of severe physical, sexual, or psychological abuse by a parent or significant other in the child's life. DID is thought to serve as a survival strategy for the child in this traumatic environment.

   C. Diagnosis/outcome identification
      1. Nursing diagnoses are formulated from the data gathered during the assessment phase and with background knowledge regarding etiological implications for the illness.
      2. Some common nursing diagnoses for clients with dissociative disorders include:
         a. Altered thought processes.
         b. Ineffective individual coping.
         c. Personal identity disturbance.
         d. Sensory-perceptual alteration.
      3. Outcome criteria are identified for measuring the effectiveness of nursing care.
   D. Planning/implementation
      1. Nursing care of the individual with a dissociative disorder is aimed at restoration of normal thought processes.
      2. Assistance is provided to the client in an effort to determine strategies for coping with stress by means other than dissociation from the environment.
   E. Evaluation is based on accomplishment of previously established outcome criteria.
   F. Medical treatment modalities for dissociative disorders
      1. Individual psychotherapy
      2. Hypnosis
      3. Supportive care
      4. **Integration** therapy (DID)

VII. Summary
VIII. Critical Thinking Exercise
VIII. Review Questions

ANSWERS TO CRITICAL THINKING EXERCISE

1. Reassurance of his safety and security.

2. Encourage him to discuss the stressful life situation that preceded the fugue state and his feelings associated with his life situation.

3. To develop more adaptive coping strategies.

CASE STUDIES FOR USE WITH STUDENT LEARNING

Case Study No. 1: Conversion Disorder

Carol has always been very shy. Her parents had been concerned about this when Carol was a child and had tried to bring her out of her shyness by involving her with other children, but were not successful. Carol preferred to be alone and seemed to be perfectly contented to be so. When Carol was in college, she took courses that she could study in solitude. The courses that required public participation often sent Carol into feelings of panic. She visited the student health center and the counseling center at the college. The student health center would provide her with medication to help her through anxious times, and the counseling center would try to help her with coping strategies to get through the anxiety. When she graduated from college, Carol got a job in the research and development department of a pharmaceutical company. It was the perfect job for Carol. She was able to do her research without much interpersonal interaction with others. However, in the last year-and-a-half, the new supervisor has decided that every 6 months, the research department staff will each present their work individually to the Board of Trustees at their semi-annual meetings. Carol panicked the first time she heard this, but with the help of some anti-anxiety medication, made it through the first presentation. When it was time for her second presentation, she woke up the morning of the meeting and was unable to speak. She presented herself at the emergency department (ED), and her boss was notified of her hospitalization. She was released when nothing physiological could be found. Today is the day of Carol's scheduled presentation. She has again awakened with the inability to make a sound. She has presented herself to the ED and does not appear to be very concerned about the problem. The admitting ED physician cannot find an organic reason for her **aphonia**. A psychiatrist is notified, and Carol is admitted to the psychiatric unit with a diagnosis of conversion disorder, aphonia. Design a care plan for Carol.

Case Study No. 2: Somatization Disorder

Lois's psychiatrist has admitted her to the psychiatric unit with a diagnosis of somatization disorder. Lois is 38 years old, and has been seeing a psychiatrist off and on since she was 16 years old, when the family was deserted by her father. Lois was the oldest of five children. At that time, Lois was admitted to the hospital by the family physician for "abdominal pain." No physical etiology was found, and the physician told Lois's mother that Lois suffered from "nervous stomach." Over the years, she has been either treated on an outpatient basis or hospitalized for chest pain, abdominal pain, backaches, food intolerances, and fatigue. She has had a hysterectomy and a thyroidectomy. She is insisting at this time that she has a problem with her stomach that the doctor is not finding. She is very depressed and tells the nurse, "I can't stand all this pain. I just can't understand why the doctor can't find my problem. I know I'm depressed, but that's not causing my stomach pain. They need to keep looking for it." The psychiatrist keeps reassuring Lois that no pathophysiology exists for her pain. Design a care plan for Lois.

LEARNING ACTIVITIES

Exercise I. BEHAVIORS ASSOCIATED WITH SOMATOFORM DISORDERS

Identify which somatoform disorder the behaviors listed are associated with. List the primary nursing diagnosis for each.
   a.   Somatization disorder
   b.   Pain Disorder
   c.   Hypochondriasis
   d.   Conversion Disorder
   e.   Body Dysmorphic Disorder

_____ 1. Nancy fell on the ice last winter and injured her elbow. She complains that she has had pain ever since, even though x-rays reveal the elbow has healed appropriately.
   Nursing diagnosis:_____

_____ 2. Virginia has some freckles across her nose and cheeks. She visits dermatologists regularly trying to find one who will "get rid of these huge spots on my skin."

Nursing diagnosis:_____

_____ 3. Franklin is assigned to secure a contract for his company. The boss tells Franklin, "If we don't get this contract, the company may have to fold." When Franklin wakes up on the morning of the negotiations, he is unable to see. The doctor has ruled out organic pathology.
Nursing diagnosis:_____

_____ 4. Sarah has had what she calls a "delicate stomach" for years. She has sought out many physicians with complaints of nausea and vomiting, abdominal pain, bloating, and diarrhea. No organic pathology can be detected.
Nursing diagnosis:_____

_____ 5. John's father died of a massive myocardial infarction when John (now age 34) was 15 years old. The two of them were playing basketball at the time. Since then, John becomes panicky when he feels his heart beating faster than usual. He takes his pulse several times a day, and seeks out a physical exam from his physician several times a year.
Nursing diagnosis:_____

Exercise II. BEHAVIORS ASSOCIATED WITH DISSOCIATIVE DISORDERS

Identify which dissociative disorder the behaviors listed are associated with.

a. Localized amnesia	e. Dissociative fugue
b. Selective amnesia	f. Dissociative identity disorder
c. Generalized amnesia	g. Depersonalization disorder
d. Continuous amnesia	

_____ 1. A young man is brought into the emergency department by the police. He does not know who he is or anything at all about his life.

_____ 2. A young man is brought into the emergency department by the police. He gives his identity and home address (which is several hundred miles away) to the admissions clerk. He tells the nurse he is very frightened, because he doesn't know when or how he came to be in this place.

_____ 3. Sandra is a clerk in an all-night convenience store. Three nights ago, the store was robbed at gunpoint, and Sandra was locked in a storage compartment for several hours until the manager was contacted by passersby who reported the robbery. She has been unable to recall the incident until just today, when details began to emerge. She is now able to report the entire event to the authorities.

_____ 4. Sam is a salesman for a leading manufacturing company. His job requires that he make presentations for large corporations who are considering Sam's company product. Sam is up for promotion, and realizes that the outcomes of these presentations will weigh heavily on whether or not he gets the promotion. Lately, he has been worried that he is going insane. Each time he is about to make a presentation, his thinking becomes "foggy," his body feels without life, and he describes the feeling as being somewhat "anesthetized." These episodes sometimes last for hours and are beginning to interfere with his performance.

_____ 5. Melody's husband complained of severe chest pain. Melody called the ambulance and accompanied her husband to the hospital. He died of a massive myocardial infarction in the emergency department. With the help of family and friends, Melody made arrangements for the memorial service and the burial. Now that it is all over, Melody is able to remember only certain aspects about the time since her husband first experienced the severe pain. She remembers the doctor telling her that her husband was dead, but she cannot remember attending the funeral service.

_____ 6. Margaret explains to the nurse that during the last year, she has had periods of time for which she cannot account. She has been attending college, and she finds pages of notes in her notebook that she cannot recall writing. Her roommate recently recounted an incident that took place when they were supposedly out together, for which Margaret has no recall. Most recently she has been hospitalized when her roommate found her unconscious in their room with an empty bottle of sleeping pills beside her. She tells the nurse she has no memory of taking the pills.

_____ 7. Kelly was involved in an automobile accident in which her best friend was killed. Kelly remembers nothing about the accident, nor does she remember anything that has occurred since the accident.

TEST QUESTIONS

1. Louise has just moved to a new city and sees her new primary care practitioner for the first time because of GI distress. When she takes Louise's history, the primary care practitioner suspects some type of somatoform disorder. What is the *next step* necessary to confirm a diagnosis in this category?
    a. GI work-up
  • b. Thorough physical examination
    c. Review of old medical records
    d. Referral to a psychiatrist

2. The primary care practitioner diagnoses Louise with somatization disorder. Which of the following data enable the physician to distinguish between hypochondriasis and somatization disorder in arriving at a diagnosis for Louise?
    a. Pain
    b. Gender distribution
  • c. Persistent fear
    d. Impaired functioning

3. Tracy is a 27-year-old woman who, after being diagnosed as having major depression, borderline personality disorder, and antisocial personality disorder in previous contacts with the mental health-care system, has recently been diagnosed with dissociative identity disorder. She has been hospitalized because one of her personalities attempted suicide. What is the *primary* consideration in planning care for Tracy?
  • a. Safety
    b. Establishing trust
    c. Awareness of all personalities
    d. Recognition of events that trigger transition between personalities

4. The primary nursing diagnosis for Tracy during *this* hospitalization is:
   a. Personal Identity Disturbance
   b. Sensory-Perceptual Alteration
   c. Altered Thought Processes
   • d. Risk for Suicide

5. Which of the following psychosocial influences has been correlated with the predisposition to asthma?
   a. Unresolved Oedipus complex
   b. Underdeveloped ego
   c. Punitive superego
   • d. Unresolved dependency needs

6. The individual with essential hypertension is thought to:
   • a. Suppress anger and hostility
   b. Fear social interactions with others
   c. Project feelings onto the environment
   d. Deny responsibility for own behavior

7. The "migraine personality" includes which of the following sets of characteristics?
   a. Highly extroverted, impulsive, and expresses anger inappropriately
   • b. Compulsive, perfectionistic, and somewhat inflexible
   c. Excessively ambitious, easily aroused hostility, and highly competitive
   d. Chronic feelings of depression and despair, and has a tendency toward self-pity

8. The individual who suffers from migraine headaches is thought to have:
   • a. Repressed anger.
   b. Suppressed anxiety.
   c. Unresolved dependency needs.
   d. Displaced aggression.

9. Anxiety is involved in understanding the problem of dissociative amnesia. The defense mechanism used in this psychogenic process is:
   a. Suppression.
   b. Denial.
   • c. Repression.

d. Rationalization.

10. Bill C. has been diagnosed with a dissociative disorder that is identified as a fugue state. Which of the following behaviors best illustrates this diagnosis?
    a. Seeking privacy in his office
    b. Driving a long distance to visit a friend
 • c. Sudden unexpected travel away from home
    d. Taking a vacation to a place he would not usually go

11. Bill's unusual activity (from question #10) may have occurred in response to which of the following?
    a. Severe psychological stress
    b. Excessive alcohol use
    c. Psychogenic amnesia
 • d. a or b

12. Which of the following is an example of systematized amnesia?
    a. George has no memory of his entire lifetime, including his personal identity.
 • b. AnnMarie knows she was beaten by her mother as a child, but cannot remember the details of any of the beatings.
    c. Nancy, who was driving the car in which her best friend was killed, cannot recall the accident or events since the accident.
    d. Sarah, whose home was destroyed in a tornado, only remembers feeling the tornado hit, hearing the ambulance siren, and waking up in the hospital.

13. **Type C personality** characteristics include all of the following *except:*
    a. exhibits a calm, placid exterior.
    b. puts others' needs before their own.
 • c. has a strong competitive drive.
    d. holds resentment toward others for perceived "wrongs."

14. Friedman and Rosenman identified two major character traits common to individuals with Type A personality They are:
 • a. excessive competitive drive and chronic sense of time urgency.
    b. unmet dependency needs and low self-esteem.
    c. chronic depression and tendency toward self-pity.
    d. self-sacrificing and perfectionistism.

15. Which of the following statements is true about Type B personality?
    a. Their personalities are the exact opposite of Type A's.
- b. They lack the need for competition and comparison as do Type A's.
    c. They are usually less successful than Type A's.
    d. They do not perform as well under pressure as Type A's.

CHAPTER 18. DISORDERS OF HUMAN SEXUALITY

CHAPTER FOCUS

The focus of this chapter is on nursing care of clients with sexual disorders. Etiological implications and symptomatology are explored, and nursing care is presented in the context of the six steps of the nursing process. Medical treatment modalities are also discussed.

LEARNING OBJECTIVES

After reading this chapter, the student will be able to:
1. Describe developmental processes associated with human sexuality.
2. Discuss historical and epidemiological aspects of paraphilias and sexual dysfunction disorders.
3. Identify various types of paraphilias and sexual dysfunction disorders.
4. Discuss etiological implications of paraphilias and sexual dysfunction disorders.
5. Formulate nursing diagnoses and goals of care for clients with sexual disorders.
6. Identify appropriate nursing interventions for clients with sexual disorders.
7. Evaluate care of clients with sexual disorders.
8. Describe various medical treatment modalities for clients with sexual disorders.
9. Discuss variations in sexual orientation.
10. Identify various types of sexually transmitted diseases and discuss the consequences of each.

KEY TERMS

anorgasmia	transsexualism
dyspareunia	voyeurism
exhibitionism	pedophilia
fetishism	premature ejaculation
frotteurism	retarded ejaculation
gonorrhea	sadism
homosexuality	sensate focus
lesbianism	syphilis
masochism	transvestic fetishism
orgasm	vaginismus
paraphilia	

CHAPTER OUTLINE/LECTURE NOTES
I. Introduction
   A. Sexuality is a basic need and an aspect of humanness that cannot be separated from life events.

B. Although not all nurses need to be educated as sex therapists, they can readily integrate information on sexuality in the care they give by focusing on preventive, therapeutic, and educational interventions to assist individuals attain, regain, or maintain sexual wellness.

II. Development of Human Sexuality
A. Birth through age 12
    1. By age 2 or 2½, children know what gender they are.
    2. By age 4 or 5, children engage in heterosexual play.
    3. Late childhood and preadolescence may be characterized by homosexual play.
    4. Ages 10 to 12 are preoccupied with pubertal changes and the beginnings of romantic interest in the opposite gender.
B. Adolescence
    1. Adolescents relate to sexual issues such as how to deal with new or more powerful sexual feelings, whether to participate in various types of sexual behavior, how to recognize love, how to prevent unwanted pregnancy, and how to define age-appropriate sex roles.
C. Adulthood. This period begins at approximately 20 years of age and continues to age 65.
    1. Marital sex. Choosing a marital partner or developing a sexual relationship with another individual is one of the major tasks in the early years of this life-cycle stage.
    2. Extramarital sex. Approximately 20 to 30 percent of men have extramarital sex at some time during their marriages compared with about 15 to 20 percent of women.
    3. Sex and the single person. Attitudes about sexual intimacy vary greatly from individual to individual. Some enjoy their freedom and independence whereas others are desperately seeking an intimate relationship.
    4. The middle years—46 to 65 years. Hormonal changes occurring during this period produce changes in sexual activity for both men and women.

III. Sexual Disorders
A. **Paraphilias:** a term used to identify repetitive or preferred sexual fantasies or behaviors that involve the preference for use of a nonhuman object, repetitive sexual activity with humans involving real or simulated suffering or humiliation, and repetitive sexual activity with nonconsenting partners.
    1. Historical aspects: at certain times in history, various sexual behaviors have been, and still are, condemned by certain social and religious sanctions.
    2. Epidemiological statistics: most paraphiliacs are men, and more than 50 percent of these individuals develop the onset of their paraphilic arousal prior to age 18.
    3. Types of paraphilias
        a. **Exhibitionism:** characterized by recurrent, intense, sexual urges, behaviors, or sexually arousing fantasies involving the exposure of one's genitals to an unsuspecting stranger.

b. **Fetishism:** involves recurrent, intense, sexual urges or behaviors or sexually arousing fantasies involving the use of nonliving objects. The objects are commonly intimately associated with the human body (for example, shoes, gloves, stockings).

c. **Frotteurism:** the recurrent preoccupation with intense sexual urges or fantasies involving touching or rubbing against a nonconsenting person.

d. **Pedophilia:** recurrent sexual urges, behaviors, or sexually arousing fantasies involving sexual activity with a prepubescent child.

e. Sexual **masochism:** recurrent, intense, sexual urges, behaviors, or sexually arousing fantasies involving acts (real, not simulated) of being humiliated, beaten, bound, or otherwise made to suffer.

f. Sexual **sadism:** recurrent, intense, sexual urges, behaviors, or sexually arousing fantasies involving acts (real, not simulated) in which the psychological or physical suffering (including humiliation) of the victim is sexually exciting to the person.

g. **Voyeurism:** recurrent, intense, sexual urges, behaviors, or sexually arousing fantasies involving the act of observing unsuspecting people, usually strangers, who are either naked, in the process of disrobing, or engaging in sexual activity.

4. Etiological implications for paraphilias

a. Biological factors. Various studies have implicated several organic factors in the etiology of paraphilias. These include abnormalities in the limbic system and the temporal lobe. Abnormal levels of androgens have also been implicated.

b. Psychoanalytical theory. Suggests that a paraphiliac is one who has failed the normal developmental process toward heterosexual adjustment. This occurs when the individual fails to resolve the Oedipal crisis and either identifies with the parent of the opposite gender or selects an inappropriate object for libido cathexis.

c. Behavioral theory. The behavioral model hypothesizes that whether or not an individual engages in paraphiliac behavior depends on the type of reinforcement he receives following the behavior. The initial act may be committed for various reasons (for example, modeling the paraphilic behavior of others or mimicking sexual behavior depicted in the media). But once the initial act has been committed, a conscious evaluation of the behavior occurs, and a choice is made of whether or not to repeat it.

d. Theoretical integration. It is most likely that the etiology of paraphilias is influenced by multiple factors.

5. Medical treatment modalities

a. Biological treatment. The focus of this treatment is on blocking or decreasing the level of circulating androgens.

b. Psychoanalytical therapy. With this type of therapy, the client is assisted to identify unresolved conflicts and traumas from early childhood, thus resolving the anxiety that prevents him or her from forming appropriate sexual relationships.

      c. Behavioral therapy. Aversion techniques, such as the use of electric shock and chemical induction of nausea and vomiting, usually in combination with exposure to photographs depicting the undesired behavior, have been used to modify undesirable paraphilic behavior.

  6. Role of the nurse

      a. Nursing may best become involving in the primary prevention process.

      b. The focus of primary prevention in sexual disorders is to intervene in home life or other facets of childhood in an effort to prevent problems from developing.

      c. An additional concern of primary prevention is to assist in the development of adaptive coping strategies to deal with stressful life situations.

B. Sexual dysfunctions

  1. Usually occur as a problem in one of the following phases of the sexual response cycle:

      a. Phase I: Desire

      b. Phase II: Excitement

      c. Phase III. **Orgasm**

      d. Phase IV. Resolution

  2. Historical and epidemiological aspects related to sexual dysfunction

      a. Concurrent with the cultural changes occurring during the sexual revolution of the 1960s and 1970s came an increase in scientific research into sexual physiology and sexual dysfunctions.

      b. Masters and Johnson pioneered this work with their studies on human sexual response and the treatment of sexual dysfunctions.

  3. Types of sexual dysfunction

      a. Sexual desire disorders

          (1) Hypoactive sexual desire disorder. Persistent or recurrent deficiency or absence of sexual fantasies and desire for sexual activity.

          (2) Sexual aversion disorder. Persistent or recurrent extreme aversion to, and avoidance of, all or almost all, genital sexual contact with a sexual partner.

      b. Sexual arousal disorders

          (1) Female sexual arousal disorder. Failure to attain, or to maintain until the completion of the sexual activity, an adequate lubrication-swelling response of sexual excitement.

          (2) Male erectile disorder. Persistent or recurrent inability to attain, or to maintain until completion of the sexual activity, an adequate erection.

      c. Orgasmic disorders

          (1) Female orgasmic disorder (**anorgasmia**). The recurrent or persistent delay in, or absence of, orgasm following a normal sexual excitement phase.

          (2) Male orgasmic disorder (**retarded ejaculation**). Persistent or recurrent delay in, or absence of, orgasm following a normal sexual excitement

phase during sexual activity that the clinician, taking into account the person's age, judges to be adequate in focus, intensity, and duration.

   (3) **Premature ejaculation.** Persistent or recurrent ejaculation with minimal sexual stimulation or before, upon, or shortly after penetration and before the person wishes it.

d. Sexual pain disorders

   (1) **Dyspareunia.** Recurrent or persistent genital pain in either a male or female before, during or after sexual intercourse, that is not associated with **vaginismus** or with lack of lubrication.

   (2) Vaginismus. An involuntary constriction of the outer one third of the vagina that prevents penile insertion and intercourse.

e. Sexual dysfunction due to a general medical condition and substance-induced sexual dysfunction

   (1) With these disorders, the sexual dysfunction is judged to be caused by the direct physiological effects of a general medical condition or use of a substance.

4. Etiological implications for sexual dysfunctions

a. Biological factors. Suggestive evidence exists of a relationship between serum testosterone and hypoactive sexual desire disorder in men and increased libido in women. Certain medications, such as antihypertensives, antipsychotics, antidepressants, anxiolytics, and anticonvulsants may also be implicated in the etiology of hypoactive sexual desire disorder. Erectile disorders in men may be affected by arteriosclerosis and diabetes. In women, consumption of alcohol, as well as certain medications, have been shown to affect a woman's ability to have orgasms. Various organic factors have also been associated with painful intercourse in both men and women.

b. Psychosocial factors. A number of psychosocial factors have been associated with sexual desire disorders, as well as with virtually all the sexual disorders. A few of these factors include religious orthodoxy, secret sexual deviations, fear of pregnancy, childhood sexual abuse, rape, fears, anxiety, and depression.

IV. Application of the Nursing Process

   A. Assessment. A tool for gathering a sexual history is included. Additional information should be gathered for the clients who have medical or surgical conditions that may affect their sexuality; clients with infertility problems, sexually transmitted disease, or complaints of sexual inadequacy; clients who are pregnant, or present with gynecological problems; those seeking information on abortion or family planning; and individuals in premarital, marital, and psychiatric counseling.

   B. Diagnosis/outcome identification

      1. Nursing diagnoses for clients experiencing sexual dysfunction include:

         a. Sexual dysfunction

         b. Altered sexuality patterns

      2. Outcome criteria are identified for measuring the effectiveness of nursing care.

C. Planning/implementation
  1. Nursing intervention for the client with sexual disorders is aimed at assisting the individual to gain or regain the aspect of his or her sexuality that is desired.
  2. The nurse must remain nonjudgmental and ensure that personal feelings, attitudes, and values have been clarified and do not interfere with acceptance of the client.
D. Client/family education
E. Evaluation is based on accomplishment of previously established outcome criteria.

V. Treatment Modalities for Sexual Dysfunctions
  A. Hypoactive sexual desire disorder
    1. Testosterone
    2. Cognitive therapy
    3. Behavioral therapy
    4. Marital therapy
  B. Sexual aversion disorder
    1. Systematic desensitization
    2. Antidepressant medication
  C. Female sexual arousal disorder
    1. **Sensate focus** exercises
  D. Male erectile disorder
    1. Sensate focus exercises
    2. Group therapy
    3. Hypnotherapy
    4. Systematic desensitization
    5. Testosterone
    6. Sildenafil (Viagra)
    7. Penile implantation
  E. Female and male orgasmic disorder
    1. Sensate focus exercises
    2. Directed masturbation training
  F. Premature ejaculation
    1. Sensate focus exercises
    2. "Squeeze" technique
  G. Dyspareunia
    1. Physical and gynecological examination
    2. Systematic desensitization
  H. Vaginismus
    1. Education of the woman and her partner regarding the anatomy and physiology of the disorder
    2. Systematic desensitization with dilators of graduated sizes

VI. Variations in Sexual Orientation
  A. **Homosexuality**. The expression of a sexual preference for individuals of the same gender. This is only seen by the psychiatric community as a problem when the

individual experiences "persistent and marked distress about his or her sexual orientation."

1. Etiological implications
    a. Biological theories. It has been suggested that a genetic tendency for homosexuality may be inherited or that a decreased level of testosterone may be influential. Neither hypothesis has been substantiated.
    b. Psychosocial theories
        (1) Freud suggested a possible fixation in the stage of development when homosexual tendencies are common.
        (2) Bieber and coworkers suggested a dysfunctional family pattern as an etiological influence in the development of male homosexuality. The mother was described as dominant, overprotective, possessive, and seductive in her interactions with her son. The father was found to be passive, distant, and covertly or overtly hostile, and was openly devalued and dominated by the mother.
2. Special concerns
    a. Sexually transmitted diseases, in particular, AIDS
    b. Discovery of their sexual orientation
    c. Fear of being rejected by parents and significant others
    d. Discrimination within society

B. **Transsexualism:** a disorder of gender identity or gender dysphoria (unhappiness or dissatisfaction with one's gender) of the most extreme variety. An individual, despite having the anatomical characteristics of a given gender, has the self-perception of being of the opposite gender.
1. Etiological implications
    a. Biological theories. There has been some speculation that gender-disordered individuals may be exposed to inappropriate hormones during the prenatal period, which can result in a genetic female having male genitals, or a genetic male having female genitals. Evidence is inconclusive.
    b. Psychosocial theories
        (1) Extensive, pervasive childhood femininity in a boy or childhood masculinity in a girl increases the likelihood of transsexualism.
        (2) Repeated cross-dressing of a young child.
        (3) Lack of separation/individuation of a boy from his mother.
2. Special concerns
    a. Extensive psychological testing is conducted prior to surgical intervention.
    b. Hormonal treatment is initiated during this period.
    c. Both men and women continue to receive maintenance hormone therapy following surgery.

C. Bisexuality: Not exclusively heterosexual or homosexual, but sexually active with members of both genders
1. Etiological implications
    a. Little research exists on the etiology of bisexuality.
    b. Freud believed that all humans are inherently bisexual.

     c. Riddle suggests that gender identity (determining whether one is heterosexual or homosexual or both) most likely continues to evolve throughout one's lifetime.

VII. Sexually Transmitted Diseases

    A. Sexually transmitted diseases (STDs) are a group of disease syndromes that can be transmitted sexually, irrespective of whether the disease has genital pathological manifestations. STDs may be transmitted from one person to another through heterosexual or homosexual, anal, oral, or genital contact.

    B. STDs are at epidemic levels in the United States.

    C. The nurse's first responsibility in STD control is to educate clients who may develop or have a sexually transmitted infection.

    D. Prevention of STDs is the ideal goal, but early detection and appropriate treatment continue to be considered a realistic objective.

    E. Information regarding the following types of STDs is presented:
       1. **Gonorrhea**
       2. **Syphilis**
       3. Chlamydial infection
       4. Genital herpes
       5. Genital warts
       6. Hepatitis B
       7. Acquired immunodeficiency syndrome (AIDS)

VIII. Summary

IX. Critical Thinking Exercise

X. Review Questions

ANSWERS TO CRITICAL THINKING EXERCISE

1. Sexual dysfunction related to unresolved sexual issues from her own teen years evidenced by loss of sexual desire.

2. Encourage her to talk about the incident from her adolescence. Encourage her to talk about her relationship with her husband. Explore her fears of having sex with her husband with the teenagers in the house. Help her problem solve ways to overcome these fears (for example, place a lock on their bedroom door). Take a medication history to ensure lack of sexual desire is not related to a substance. Suggest they spend regular time alone (away from the house if necessary). Help her problem solve ways to accomplish this. Help her to understand that she and her husband need not return to the level of sexual interaction in which they participated early in their marriage.

3. To resume sexual activity with her husband at a level of participation that is satisfactory to both. (This may mean that her husband will have to compromise his level of sexual desire. If they are unable to resolve their differences, the nurse may need to make a referral to a sex therapist who specializes in this type of problem.)

LEARNING ACTIVITY

VALUES CLARIFICATION

Answer the following questions. Move into small groups and analyze and discuss your answers.

1. As a child, when was the first time you discussed sex? With whom?

2. As an adolescent, when was the first time you began to notice a change in your body? Were you proud of it? Did you want to change it in any way?

3. Did your parents talk to you outright about sex? If not, what was the underlying message?

4. Did you make an active decision to become sexually active, or did it happen spontaneously? Has "safe sex" become an important consideration?

5. What are your feelings about sex between elderly individuals?

6. Describe your tolerance of homosexuality as a variation in sexual orientation.

7. Describe your tolerance of a homosexual man as your fifth grade son's teacher.

8. You discover your 10-year-old sister and her two playmates playing "doctor" in the garage. What is your response?

In your opinion,

9. Should a married woman, who has a satisfactory sexual relationship with her husband, masturbate with a vibrator?

10. Do most parents give their daughters as much sexual freedom as they do their sons? Should they?

11. Do parents who give contraceptives to their adolescents present a message that having sex is okay?

12. Are individuals who have sex change operations freaks?

13. Does pornography lead to sexual crimes?

14. Are oral and anal sex deviant behaviors?

15. Do you ever have the right to refuse treatment to an AIDS client?

TEST QUESTIONS

1. Tom and Susan are seeking treatment at the sex therapy clinic. They have been married for 3 years. Susan was a virgin when they married. She admits that she has never really enjoyed sex, but lately has developed an aversion to it. They have not had sexual intercourse for about 5 months. Sexual history reveals that Susan grew up in a family who was very closed about sexual issues with the implication that sex was

sinful and dirty. The physician would most likely assign which of the following diagnoses to Susan?
   a. Dyspareunia
   b. Vaginismus
   c. Anorgasmia
 • d. Sexual aversion disorder

2. The most appropriate nursing diagnosis for Susan would be:
   a. Pain related to vaginal constriction.
 • b. Sexual dysfunction related to negative teachings about sex.
   c. Altered sexuality patterns related to lack of desire for sex.
   d. Self-esteem disturbance related to inability to please her husband sexually.

3. Which of the following interventions by the nurse may initiate treatment for Tom and Susan?
 • a. Assessing client's perception of the problem
   b. Initiating sensate focus exercises
   c. Initiating directed masturbation training
   d. Teaching the "squeeze" technique

4. The sex therapist assigned to the case would likely choose which of the following therapies for Susan?
   a. Sensate focus exercises
 • b. Systematic desensitization
   c. Hypnotherapy
   d. Gradual dilation of the vagina

5. Additional therapy may include:
   a. Minor tranquilizers
   b. Group therapy
 • c. Tricyclic antidepressant
   d. Injections of testosterone

The following questions are related to paraphilias.

6. Achieving sexual satisfaction by touching or rubbing against a nonconsenting person is known as:
 • a. Frotteurism.
   b. Fetishism.

      c. Voyeurism.
      d. Sexual masochism.

7. Sexual sadists achieve satisfaction by:
      a. Being psychologically or physically abused.
•   b. Causing psychological or physical suffering to another.
      c. Engaging in sexual activity with a prepubescent child.
      d. Exposing their genitals to an unsuspecting stranger.

8. The role of the nurse in intervention with the paraphiliac is best accomplished during:
•   a. Primary prevention of the disorder.
      b. Diagnosis of the disorder.
      c. Treatment of the disorder.
      d. The rehabilitation phase of treatment.

CHAPTER 19. EATING DISORDERS

CHAPTER FOCUS

The focus of this chapter is on nursing care of clients with eating disorders. Etiological implications and symptomatology are explored, and nursing care is presented in the context of the six steps of the nursing process. Medical treatment modalities are also discussed.

LEARNING OBJECTIVES

After reading this chapter, the student will be able to:
1. Identify and differentiate among the various eating disorders.
2. Discuss epidemiological statistics related to eating disorders.
3. Describe symptomatology associated with anorexia nervosa, bulimia nervosa, and obesity, and use the information in client assessment.
4. Identify etiological implications in the development of eating disorders.
5. Formulate nursing diagnoses and goals of care for clients with eating disorders.
6. Describe appropriate interventions for behaviors associated with eating disorders.
7. Identify topics for client and family teaching relevant to eating disorders.
8. Evaluate the nursing care of clients with eating disorders.
9. Discuss various modalities relevant to treatment of eating disorders.

KEY TERMS

amenorrhea
binging
purging
body image
emaciated
anorexia
obesity
anorexigenics

CHAPTER OUTLINE/LECTURE NOTES

I. Introduction
  A. The hypothalamus contains the appetite regulation center within the brain. It regulates the body's ability to recognize when it is hungry and when it has been sated.
  B. Eating behaviors are influenced by society and culture.
  C. Historically, society and culture also have influenced what is considered desirable in the female body.
II. Epidemiological Factors

A. The incidence rate of **anorexia** nervosa among young women in the United States is approximately 14 per 100,000 population.

B. Anorexia nervosa occurs predominantly in females ages 12 to 30 years.

C. Bulimia nervosa is more prevalent than anorexia nervosa. Estimates range from 1 to 3 percent of young women.

D. Onset of bulimia nervosa occurs in late adolescence or early adulthood, with a mean age of onset of 18 years.

E. **Obesity** has been defined as a body mass index (weight/height^2) of 30 or greater.

F. Approximately 24 percent of adult males and 27 percent of adult females in the United States suffer from obesity.

III. Application of the Nursing Process

    A. Background assessment data (symptomatology)

        1. Anorexia nervosa

            a. Characterized by a morbid fear of obesity.

            b. Symptoms include gross distortion of **body image,** preoccupation with food, and refusal to eat.

            c. Weight loss is extreme, usually more than 15 percent of expected weight.

            d. Other symptoms include hypothermia, bradycardia, hypotension, edema, lanugo, and a variety of metabolic changes.

            e. **Amenorrhea** is typical and may even precede significant weight loss.

            f. There may be an obsession with food.

            g. Feelings of anxiety and depression are common.

        2. Bulimia nervosa

            a. Bulimia is the episodic, uncontrolled, compulsive, rapid ingestion of large quantities of food over a short period of time (**binging**), followed by inappropriate compensatory behaviors to rid the body of the excess calories (self-induced vomiting, or the misuse of laxatives, diuretics, or enemas).

            b. Fasting or excessive exercise may also occur.

            c. Most bulimics are within a normal weight range, some slightly underweight, some slightly overweight.

            d. Excessive vomiting and laxative/diuretic abuse may lead to problems with dehydration and electrolyte imbalance.

            e. Depression, anxiety, and substance abuse are not uncommon.

        3. Etiological implications for anorexia nervosa and bulimia nervosa

            a. Biological influences

                (1) Genetics. A hereditary predisposition to eating disorders has been hypothesized. Anorexia nervosa is more common among sisters and mothers of those with the disorder than among the general population.

                (2) Neuroendocrine abnormalities. Some speculation has occurred regarding a primary hypothalamic dysfunction in anorexia nervosa.

            b. Psychodynamic theory suggests that eating disorders result from very early and profound disturbances in mother-infant interactions, resulting in retarded ego development and an unfulfilled sense of separation-individuation.

  c. Family influences
   (1) Conflict avoidance. Families may promote and maintain psychosomatic symptoms, including anorexia nervosa, in an effort to avoid spousal conflict. The sick child becomes the problem, and focus on the conflict is diverted.
   (2) Elements of power and control. Power and control may become the overriding elements in the family of the client with an eating disorder. Parental criticism promotes an increase in obsessive and perfectionistic behavior on the part of the child, who continues to seek love, approval, and recognition. Ambivalence toward the parents develops, and distorted eating patterns may represent a rebellion against the parents—a way to gain control.
 4. Obesity
  a. A body mass index (weight divided by height squared) of 30 is considered obesity.
  b. At this level, weight alone can contribute to increases in morbidity and mortality.
  c. Obese people are at higher risk for hyperlipidemia, diabetes mellitus, osteoarthritis, angina, and respiratory insufficiency.
 5. Etiological implications for obesity
  a. Biological influences
   (1) Genetics. Eighty percent of children born of two obese parents will also be obese. Twin studies have also supported a hereditary factor.
   (2) Physiological factors
    (a) Lesions in the appetite and satiety centers of the hypothalamus
    (b) Hypothyroidism
    (c) Decreased insulin production
    (d) Increased cortisone production
   (3) Lifestyle factors
    (a) Increased caloric intake
    (b) Sedentary lifestyle
  b. Psychosocial influences
   (1) Unresolved dependency needs
   (2) Fixation in the oral stage of psychosexual development
B. Diagnosis/outcome identification
 1. Nursing diagnoses for the client with eating disorders include:
  a. Imbalanced nutrition: less than body requirements.
  b. Deficient fluid volume (risk for or actual).
  c. Ineffective denial.
  d. Imbalanced nutrition: more than body requirements.
  e. Body image/self-esteem disturbance.
  f. Anxiety (moderate to severe).
 2. Outcome criteria are identified for measuring the effectiveness of nursing care.
C. Planning/implementation

1. Nursing care of the client with an eating disorder is aimed at restoring nutritional balance.
2. Emphasis is also placed on helping the client gain control over life situations in ways other than inappropriate eating behaviors.
3. Self-esteem and positive self-image are promoted in ways that relate to aspects other than appearance.

D. Client/family education
E. Evaluation is based on accomplishment of previously established outcome criteria.

IV. Treatment Modalities
   A. Behavior modification
   B. Individual therapy
   C. Family therapy
   D. Psychopharmacology

V. Summary
VI. Critical Thinking Exercise
VII. Review Questions

ANSWERS TO CRITICAL THINKING EXERCISE

1. Restoring her nutritional condition.
2. A program of behavior modification, with privileges based on weight gain
3. The door to her bathroom will need to be kept locked for at least 1 hour following meals. However, she will still need to be watched carefully because she may go into other clients' bathrooms to purge herself.

CASE STUDY FOR USE WITH STUDENT LEARNING

Case Study: Bulimia Nervosa

Abby, age, 29, was married and the mother of a 5-year-old girl. Her husband, Tom, was a rising young executive in a prominent business firm. Abby did not work outside the home, and Tom had expectations about how he expected Abby to care for their daughter and their home. Abby had grown up as the only child of a professional couple who had high expectations of her. Feeling unable to measure up to their expectations, Abby had developed anorexia nervosa during her sophomore year in high school, and the family had spent several years in family therapy. Abby went to college in a distant city. During these years, she did not go home often. She joined a sorority, but often felt as though she did not quite fit in with these young women. She felt very flattered when Tom began to pay attention to her during her junior year in college. But she continued to feel anxious and insecure, and during these periods of anxiety, Abby would resort to maladaptive eating patterns to cope. During this time, however, the eating behavior more often took the form of binging. She would eat whole boxes of cookies, cakes, or candy, followed by periods of intense depression. In order to keep from gaining weight, she would self-induce vomiting, or take massive doses of laxatives. She exercised excessively. She managed to keep her weight within normal limits, while hiding her behavior from her boyfriend and classmates. Once she and Tom were married, some of the anxiety subsided, and she relied less on the maladaptive eating behaviors. However, lately, she has been called upon by her husband to entertain business associates, which has created a great deal of anxiety for Abby. Tom tells her exactly how he expects things to be and also tells her how much her appearance and behavior affects how these business associates will view them. She feels a great deal of pressure from Tom to be "the perfect wife" and just doesn't feel she can measure up. She has begun to binge and purge daily. Last night, she was binging after Tom and their daughter had gone to bed. Tom heard her vomiting in their bathroom. He got up to investigate and found her leaning over the toilet, in which he noted a large amount of blood. He took her to the emergency room where she was treated for a bleeding esophageal varicosity. She was stabilized and admitted to the psychiatric unit. Diagnosis: Bulimia Nervosa. Design a care plan for Abby.

LEARNING ACTIVITY

Check the eating disorder to which the symptoms in the left-hand column apply. Some may apply to more than one disorder. The first is completed as an example.

Symptoms	Anorexia Nervosa	Bulimia Nervosa	Obesity
1. Depression	X	X	
2. Amenorrhea			
3. Risk of diabetes mellitus			
4. Erosion of tooth enamel			
5. Preoccupation with food			
6. Self-induced vomiting			
7. Fixed in oral stage of development			
8. Is markedly underweight			
9. Weight is close to normal			
10. Is markedly overweight			
11. Abuse of substances is not uncommon			
12. May be related to hypothyroidism			
13. May be related to issues of control			

14. Genetics may play a role in the cause			
15. Takes in enormous amounts of food without gaining weight			

TEST QUESTIONS

Situation: Stephanie, age 23, calls the eating disorders clinic for an appointment. She tells the nurse who does the assessment interview that she was hospitalized and diagnosed with anorexia nervosa when she was 14 years old. Since that time, she has seen a therapist periodically when she feels her anxiety is increasing and the fear of eating starts to take hold. She recently graduated from college and moved to this city, where she began a new job as a production assistant at a local TV station. She is nervous about starting the new job, and wants to "do a perfect job, so I can move up quickly to a more challenging position." She tells the nurse that she has been taking laxatives every day, and some days after eating, she will self-induce vomiting. She knows this is not good but feels powerless to stop. She is 5′6″ tall and weighs 105 lb.

1. What other physical manifestations might the nurse expect to find upon assessment?
   a. High blood pressure, fever
   • b. Low blood pressure, low temperature
   c. Slow heart rate, fever
   d. Fast heart rate, low blood pressure

2. The *primary* nursing diagnosis on which the nurse will base her plan of care is:
   a. Ineffective denial
   b. Body image disturbance
   c. Self-esteem disturbance
   • d. Imbalanced nutrition, less than body requirements

3. What other therapy might the physician prescribe?
   • a. Fluoxetine (Prozac)
   b. Diazepam (Valium)
   c. Fenfluramine (Pondimin)
   d. Meprobamate (Equanil)

Situation: Betty, a 38-year-old woman, is also being followed in the eating disorders clinic. Betty is 5′4″ and weighs 250 pounds. When she first came to the clinic 2 years ago, she weighed 347 pounds. Her diagnosis at that time was morbid obesity. The dietitian put her on a 1500 calorie/day diet and the physician at the clinic prescribed fenfluramine and phentermine, the "fen-fen" drugs that were so popular at that time. Since then, fenfluramine has been taken off the market because it caused pulmonary hypertension in a number of individuals. Betty says to the nurse, "I don't know what to do! I know I can't lose weight without those drugs. That's the only reason I lost any at all. And I've already gained some back since I quit taking them!"

4. Fenfluramine and phentermine are part of which of the following classifications of drugs?
   a. Antidepressants
   - b. Anorexigenics
   c. Antianxiety
   d. Anticonvulsants

5. The nurse explains to Betty that the physician may be able to prescribe another medication to help her lose weight. Which of the following might the nurse expect the physician to prescribe?
   a. Diazepam (Valium)
   b. Dexfenfluramine (Redux)
   - c. Sibutramine (Meridia)
   d. Pemoline (Cylert)

6. The nurse tells Betty that she will lose weight even without medication if she just sticks to her diet and adds some exercise to her routine. What would be the most appropriate exercise for the nurse to suggest for Betty?
   a. Low-impact aerobics 3 times a week
   b. Jogging ½ mile twice a week
   c. Swimming at the YWCA 30 minutes/day
   - d. Walking around her neighborhood for 20 minutes/day (weather permitting)

General questions related to eating disorders:

7. The best approach to establish adequate eating patterns in a client with anorexia nervosa is to assume a positive expectation of the client. Which is the best statement by the nurse?
   a. "I'll give you a 1-hour time limit."
   b. "I will allow you space to eat in private."
   - c. "I will sit quietly with you while you eat."
   d. "There are people who would truly appreciate the food that you waste."

8. If an anorectic client is being forced to eat, it is important for the nurse to implement which one of the following interventions?

a. Use praise or flattery for adequate intake
b. Discuss eating behaviors and what is considered appropriate
c. Provide three large meals daily with between meal snacks
• d. Observe bathroom behavior following meals

9. Assessment of an anorectic client is likely to reveal which of the following?
   • a. Amenorrhea
   b. Hypertension
   c. Tachycardia
   d. Hyperthermia

10. Assessment of a bulimic client is likely to reveal which of the following?
    a. Weight loss in excess of 15% of expected weight
    b. Amenorrhea
    • c. Electrolyte imbalance
    d. Hypertension

CHAPTER 20. PERSONALITY DISORDERS

CHAPTER FOCUS

The focus of this chapter is on nursing care of clients with personality disorders. Etiological implications and symptomatology are explored, and nursing care is presented in the context of the six steps of the nursing process. Medical treatment modalities are also discussed.

LEARNING OBJECTIVES

After reading this chapter, the student will be able to:
1. Define *personality*.
2. Compare stages of personality development according to Sullivan, Erikson, and Mahler.
3. Identify various types of personality disorders.
4. Discuss historical and epidemiological statistics related to various personality disorders.
5. Describe symptomatology associated with borderline personality disorder and antisocial personality disorder, and use these data in client assessment.
6. Identify etiological implications for borderline personality disorder and antisocial personality disorder.
7. Formulate nursing diagnoses and goals of care for clients with borderline personality disorder and antisocial personality disorder.
8. Describe appropriate nursing interventions for behaviors associated with borderline personality disorder and antisocial personality disorder.
9. Evaluate nursing care of clients with borderline personality disorder and antisocial personality disorder.
10. Discuss various modalities relevant to treatment of personality disorders.

KEY TERMS

histrionic
narcissism
object constancy
passive-aggressive
personality
schizoid
schizotypal
splitting

CHAPTER OUTLINE/LECTURE NOTES

I. Introduction

Copyright © 2002, F. A. Davis Company

A. **Personality** is defined as a person's characteristic totality of emotional and behavioral traits apparent in ordinary life, a totality that is usually stable and predictable.

B. Personality traits are enduring patterns of perceiving, relating to, and thinking about the environment and oneself that are exhibited in a wide range of social and personal contexts.

C. Personality disorders occur when these traits become inflexible and maladaptive and cause either significant functional impairment or subjective distress.

II. Historical Aspects

  A. The first recognition that personality disorders, apart from psychosis, were cause for their own special concern was in 1801, with the recognition that an individual can behave irrationally even when the powers of intellect are intact.

  B. Personality disorders have been categorized into three clusters, according to the type of behavior observed.

    1. Cluster A: behaviors that are described as odd or eccentric

      a. Paranoid personality disorder

      b. **Schizoid** personality disorder

      c. **Schizotypal** personality disorder

    2. Cluster B: behaviors that are described as dramatic, emotional, or erratic

      a. Antisocial personality disorder

      b. Borderline personality disorder

      c. **Histrionic** personality disorder

      d. Narcissistic personality disorder

    3. Cluster C: behaviors that are described as anxious or fearful

      a. Avoidant personality disorder

      b. Dependent personality disorder

      c. Obsessive-compulsive personality disorder

III. Types of Personality Disorders

  A. Paranoid personality disorder

    1. Definition and epidemiological statistics

      a. A pattern of behavior, beginning by early adulthood and present in a variety of contexts, of pervasive distrust and suspiciousness of others such that their motives are interpreted as malevolent.

      b. The disorder is more common in men than in women.

    2. Clinical picture

      a. They are constantly on guard, hypervigilant, and ready for any real or imagined threat. They trust no one and are constantly testing the honesty of others.

      b. They are insensitive to the feelings of others but are themselves extremely oversensitive and tend to misinterpret even minute cues within the environment, magnifying and distorting them into thoughts of trickery and deception.

    3. Etiological implications

      a. Possible genetic link

      b. Subject to early parental antagonism and aggression

B. Schizoid personality disorder
   1. Definition and epidemiological statistics
      a. Characterized primarily by a profound defect in the ability to form personal relationships or to respond to others in any meaningful, emotional way.
      b. Prevalence within the general population has been estimated at between 3 and 7.5 percent, and diagnosis occurs more frequently in men that it does in women.
   2. Clinical picture
      a. They are indifferent to others, aloof, detached, and unresponsive to praise, criticism, or any other feelings expressed by others.
      b. They have no close friends and prefer to be alone. In the presence of others, they appear shy, anxious, or uneasy.
   3. Etiological implications
      a. Possible hereditary factor
      b. Childhood has been characterized as bleak, cold, unempathic, and notably lacking in nurturing.
C. Schizotypal personality disorder
   1. Definition and epidemiological statistics
      a. A graver form of the pathologically less severe schizoid personality pattern.
      b. Recent studies indicate that approximately 3 percent of the population have this disorder.
   2. Clinical picture
      a. Individuals with schizotypal personalities are aloof and isolated and behave in a bland and apathetic manner.
      b. Symptoms include magical thinking, ideas of reference, illusions, depersonalization, superstitiousness, bizarre speech, delusions, hallucinations, and withdrawal into the self.
   3. Etiological implications
      a. Possible hereditary factor
      b. Possible physiological influence, such as anatomic deficits or neurochemical dysfunctions within certain areas of the brain
      c. Early family dynamics characterized by indifference, impassivity, or formality, leading to a pattern of discomfort with personal affection and closeness
D. Antisocial personality disorder
   1. Definition and epidemiological statistics
      a. A pattern of socially irresponsible, exploitative, and guiltless behavior, evident in the tendency to fail to conform to the law, to sustain consistent employment, to exploit and manipulate others for personal gain, to deceive, and to fail to develop stable relationships
      b. Prevalence estimates in the United States range from 3 percent in men to about 1 percent in women.
   2. Clinical picture and etiological implications: presented later in this outline.

E. Borderline personality disorder
   1. Definition and epidemiological statistics
      a. Characterized by a pattern of intense and chaotic relationships, with affective instability, fluctuating and extreme attitudes regarding other people, impulsivity, directly and indirectly self-destructive behavior, and lack of a clear or certain sense of identity, life plan, or values.
      b. Prevalence estimates range from 2 percent to 3 percent of the population.
   2. Clinical picture and etiological implications: presented later in this outline.
F. Histrionic personality disorder
   1. Definition and epidemiological statistics
      a. Characterized by colorful, dramatic, and extroverted behavior in excitable, emotional persons
      b. Prevalence is thought to be about 2 to 3 percent, and it is more common in women than it is in men.
   2. Clinical picture
      a. They are self-dramatizing, attention-seeking, overly gregarious, seductive, manipulative, exhibitionistic, shallow, frivolous, labile, vain, and demanding.
      b. Highly distractible, difficulty paying attention to detail, easily influenced by others, difficulty forming close relationships, and may complain of physical symptoms.
   3. Etiological implications
      a. Possible ease of sympathetic arousal, adrenal hyperreactivity, and neurochemical imbalances
      b. Possible hereditary factor
      c. Learned behavior patterns
G. Narcissistic personality disorder
   1. Definition and epidemiological statistics
      a. Characterized by an exaggerated sense of self-worth
      b. The disorder is more common in men than it is in women.
   2. Clinical picture
      a. They are overly self-centered and exploit others in an effort to fulfill their own desires.
      b. Mood, which is often grounded in grandiosity, is usually optimistic, relaxed, cheerful, and carefree. Mood can easily change because of fragile self-esteem.
   3. Etiological implications. Family dynamics may have fostered feelings of omnipotence and grandiosity through total indulgence of the child.
H. Avoidant personality disorder
   1. Definition and epidemiological statistics
      a. Characterized by extreme sensitivity to rejection, and social withdrawal
      b. Prevalence is between 0.5 and 1 percent, and is equally common in men and women.
   2. Clinical picture

     a. They are awkward and uncomfortable in social situations. They desire to have close relationships but cannot help believing that such will result in pain and disillusionment.

     b. They may be perceived by others as timid, withdrawn, or perhaps cold and strange.

     c. They are often lonely, and express feelings of being unwanted. They view others as critical, betraying, and humiliating.

  3. Etiological implications

     a. Possible hereditary influence

     b. Parental rejection and criticism

I. Dependent personality disorder

  1. Definition and epidemiological statistics

     a. A pattern of relying excessively on others for emotional support, advice, and reassurance.

     b. The disorder is relatively common within the population. It is more common among women than men and more common in the youngest children of a family than the older ones.

  2. Clinical picture

     a. They have a notable lack of self-confidence that is often apparent in their posture, voice, and mannerisms. They are typically passive and acquiescent to the desires of others.

     b. They avoid positions of responsibility and become anxious when forced into them.

     c. They have low self-worth and are easily hurt by criticism and disapproval.

  3. Etiological implications

     a. Possible hereditary influence

     b. Stimulation and nurturance are experienced exclusively from one source, and a singular attachment is made by the infant to the exclusion of all others.

J. Obsessive-compulsive personality disorder

  1. Definition and epidemiological statistics

     a. Characterized by inflexibility about the way in which things must be done and a devotion to productivity at the exclusion of personal pleasure.

     b. The disorder is relatively common and occurs more often in men than in women. Within the family constellation, it appears to be most common in oldest children.

  2. Clinical picture

     a. They are especially concerned with matters of organization and efficiency and tend to be rigid and unbending about rules and procedures.

     b. Social behavior tends to be polite and formal.

     c. They are very "rank conscious." They can be very ingratiating with authority figures, but quite autocratic and condemnatory with subordinates.

d. On the surface, these individuals appear to be very calm and controlled, whereas underneath there is a great deal of ambivalence, conflict, and hostility.
  3. Etiological implications: overcontrol by parents, with notable lack of positive reinforcement for acceptable behavior and frequent punishment for undesirable behavior.
K. **Passive-aggressive** personality disorder
  1. Definition and epidemiological statistics
    a. A pervasive pattern of negativistic attitudes and passive resistance to demands for adequate performance in social and occupational situations.
    b. The disorder is apparently quite common, although no statistics exist that speak to its prevalence.
  2. Clinical picture
    a. They are passively resistant to authority, demands, obligations, and responsibilities by such behaviors as dawdling, procrastination, and "forgetting."
    b. They tend to be complaining, irritable, whining, argumentative, scornful, critical, discontented, disillusioned, and disgruntled.
    c. They do not acknowledge or express their anger directly, preferring instead to express it through resistant and negativistic behavior.
  3. Etiological implications: contradictory parental attitudes and inconsistent training methods
IV. Application of the Nursing Process
A. Borderline personality disorder
  1. Background assessment data
    a. Designated as "borderline" because of the tendency of these clients to fall on the border between neuroses and psychoses
    b. A pervasive pattern of instability of interpersonal relationships, self-image, and affects, and marked impulsivity beginning by early adulthood and present in a variety of contexts
    c. They are most strikingly identified by the intensity and instability of their affect and behavior.
    d. Common behaviors include:
      (1) Chronic depression.
      (2) Inability to be alone.
      (3) Clinging and distancing behaviors.
      (4) **Splitting.**
      (5) Manipulation.
      (6) Self-destructive behaviors.
      (7) Impulsivity.
    e. Etiological implications: According to Margaret Mahler's Theory of Object Relations, the individual with borderline personality disorder becomes fixed in the rapprochement phase of development (16 to 24 months). The child fails to achieve the task of autonomy.
  2. Diagnosis/outcome intervention

a. Nursing diagnoses for the client with borderline personality disorder may include:

    (1) Risk for self-mutilation.

    (2) Dysfunctional grieving.

    (3) Impaired social interaction.

    (4) Personal identity disturbance.

    (5) Anxiety (severe to panic).

    (6) Self-esteem disturbance.

b. Outcome criteria are identified for measuring the effectiveness of nursing care.

3. Planning/implementation

    a. Nursing intervention for the client with borderline personality disorder is aimed at protection of the client from self-mutilation.

    b. The nurse also seeks to assist the client to advance in the development of personality by confronting his or her true source of internalized anger.

4. Evaluation is based on accomplishment of previously established outcome criteria.

B. Antisocial personality disorder

1. Background assessment data

    a. Sometimes called sociopathic or psychopathic behavior

    b. Usually only seen in clinical settings when they are admitted by court order for psychological evaluation

    c. Most frequently encountered in prisons, jails, and rehabilitation services

    d. Common behaviors include:

        (1) Exploitation and manipulation of others for personal gain.

        (2) Belligerent and argumentative.

        (3) Lacking remorse.

        (4) Unable to delay gratification.

        (5) Low tolerance for frustration.

        (6) Inconsistent work or academic performance.

        (7) Failure to conform to societal norms.

        (8) Impulsive and reckless.

        (9) Inability to function as a responsible parent.

        (10) Inability to form lasting monogamous relationship.

    e. Etiological implications

        (1) Possible genetic influence

        (2) Having a sociopathic or alcoholic father

        (3) Behavior disordered as a child

        (4) Parental deprivation during the first 5 years of life

        (5) Inconsistent parenting

        (6) History of severe physical abuse

        (7) Extreme poverty

2. Diagnosis/outcome identification

    a. Nursing diagnoses for the client with antisocial personality disorder may include:

(1) Risk for violence toward others.

(2) Defensive coping.

(3) Self-esteem disturbance.

(4) Impaired social interaction.

(5) Knowledge deficit.

    b. Outcome criteria are identified for measuring the effectiveness of nursing care.

   3. Planning/implementation

    a. Nursing intervention for the client with antisocial personality disorder is aimed at protection of others from the client's aggression and hostility.

    b. The nurse also seeks to assist the client to delay gratification by setting limits on unacceptable behavior.

   4. Evaluation is based on accomplishment of previously established outcome criteria.

V. Treatment Modalities for Clients with Personality Disorders

   A. Interpersonal psychotherapy

   B. Psychoanalytical psychotherapy

   C. Milieu or group therapy

   D. Cognitive/behavioral therapy

   E. Psychopharmacology

VI. Summary

VII. Critical Thinking Exercises

VIII. Review Questions

ANSWERS TO CRITICAL THINKING EXERCISES

1. Even though the nurse believes Lana's declaration is untrue, she must proceed as though it is. Lana will undergo institutional procedures for overdose management with Desyrel (usually includes emesis or gastric lavage, activated charcoal, IV fluids, monitoring of vital signs, and EKG).

2. Risk for self-directed violence related to fears of abandonment.

3. Ensure that Lana is assigned various nurses to care for her (and not always the same one to which she may "cling"). Maintain consistency of care; that is, be sure that ALL nurses follow established limits and consequences with Lana and that Lana is not allowed to manipulate some nurses into violating the limits without consequences. This is Lana's way of splitting.

CASE STUDY FOR USE WITH STUDENT LEARNING

Case Study: Borderline Personality Disorder

Nancy, age 23, has just been hospitalized after she reported to her college roommate, Carol, that she had swallowed a bottle of aspirin. She has been stabilized in the ED and has been admitted to the psychiatric unit. This is Nancy's 3rd hospitalization for similar behavior since age 15. Nancy reports that her parents were divorced when she was 3 years old. She has not seen her father since that time. She lived with her mother until she was 6 years old; then her mother left her with her grandmother and went to "seek fame and fortune" in Hollywood. She sees her mother rarely. Nancy's roommate tells the admitting nurse that Nancy has been a "nervous" person ever since she has known her. "She has mood swings, and the smallest things will set her off. Once when she was particularly 'down,' I walked in on her sitting on her bed. It looked like she was cutting her arm with a razor blade. When I confronted her about it, she denied it. But I saw the blood. It really freaked me out!" Nancy's boyfriend recently broke up with her. Nancy has had a succession of boyfriends since high school. All of her relationships are very intense, and she becomes hysterical and then despondent when a boy breaks off his relationship with her. Her previous hospitalizations have been in response to these breakups. Physical exam is unremarkable except for visible scars on the underside of both upper arms. Diagnosis: Axis I: Major Depression; Axis II: Borderline Personality Disorder.

LEARNING ACTIVITY

Match the personality disorder listed on the left that is most commonly associated with the behaviors described on the right.

_____ 1. Paranoid personality disorder	a. Shows no remorse for exploitation and manipulation of others.
_____ 2. Schizoid personality disorder	b. Accepts a job he does not want to do, then does a poor job and delays past the deadline.
_____ 3. Schizotypal personality disorder	c. Believes she is entitled to special privileges others do not deserve.
_____ 4. Antisocial personality disorder	d. They are suspicious of all others with whom they come in contact.
_____ 5. Borderline personality disorder	e. Swallows a bottle of pills after therapist leaves on vacation.
_____ 6. Histrionic personality disorder	f. Believes he has a "sixth sense" and can know what others are thinking.
_____ 7. Narcissistic personality disorder	g. Allows others to make all her important decisions for her.
_____ 8. Avoidant personality disorder	h. Refuses to enter into a relationship because of fear of rejection.
_____ 9. Dependent personality disorder	i. Demonstrates highly emotional and overly dramatic behaviors.
_____ 10. Obsessive-compulsive personality disorder	j. Has a lifelong pattern of social withdrawal.
_____ 11. Passive-aggressive personality disorder	k. Believes everyone must follow the rules and that the rules can be "bent" for no one…ever.

TEST QUESTIONS

Situation: Claudia is a 27-year-old woman who has been married and divorced four times. She is admitted to the Psychiatric Unit with a diagnosis of Borderline Personality Disorder.

1. Which of the following behavior patterns best describes someone with borderline personality disorder?
    a. Social isolation
    b. Suspiciousness of others
    c. Belligerent and argumentative
    • d. Emotional instability

2. As Nancy Nurse starts to leave the unit at the end of her shift, Claudia runs up to her, puts her arms around her, and yells, "Please don't go! You're the only one who understands me. If you go, I won't have anyone!" This is an example of what type of behavior common to individuals with borderline personality disorder?
    a. Distancing
    b. Manipulation
    • c. Splitting
    d. Impulsivity

3. Which of the following nursing interventions is appropriate to help prevent the behavior described in the previous question?
    a. Put Claudia on room restriction each time it happens.
    b. Ignore such behaviors so that they will be extinguished for lack of reinforcement.
    c. Secure a verbal contract with Claudia that she will discontinue this type of behavior.
    • d. Ensure that various staff members are rotated to work with Claudia while she is in the hospital.

Situation: Joe is a client of the Psychiatric Day Treatment Program. He has been referred by his probation officer for treatment after an arrest for driving under the influence (DUI) of substances. Joe has a history of many arrests for assault, grand larceny, and other serious crimes, and has served two prison sentences. His diagnosis is Antisocial Personality Disorder.

4. Which of the following quotes is Joe's most probable comment on his past behavior?

- a. "It's not my fault."
  - b. "I'm too ashamed to talk about it."
  - c. "I just don't remember doing it."
  - d. "I'm really sorry about all the people I've hurt."

5. When he arrives on the unit for the day's activities, Joe says to the nurse, "Wow, you look great today! I'm so glad you're on duty today. You're the best nurse who works here, you know." This comment of Joe's is an example of what type of behavior commonly associated with Antisocial Personality Disorder?
   - a. Impulsivity
   - b. Manipulation
   - c. Exploitation of others
   - d. Inability to delay gratification

6. Which of the following therapies is considered *best* for the client with Antisocial Personality Disorder?
   - a. Milieu therapy
   - b. Family therapy
   - c. Individual psychotherapy
   - d. Pharmacological therapy

The following questions relate to personality disorders in general.

7. Which of the following would be typical of an individual with schizoid personality disorder?
   - a. Receiving a paper cut, Linda yells, "Help me, quick! I'm bleeding! Somebody call 911!"
   - b. Andrew becomes suspicious when John, who had an extra new year's calendar, left it on Andrew's desk as a gift.
   - c. Fred works long hours in a solitary environment, lives alone, has no friends, and seldom speaks to others.
   - d. "How dare you, a brand new employee, suggest we make these changes! We've always done it this way, and we will continue to do it this way! Those are the rules and they'll *not* be broken!"

8. Which of the following would be typical of an individual with histrionic personality disorder?
   - a. Receiving a paper cut, Linda yells, "Help me, quick! I'm bleeding! Somebody call 911!"

b. Andrew becomes suspicious when John, who had an extra new year's calendar, left it on Andrew's desk as a gift.
c. Fred works long hours in a solitary environment, lives alone, has no friends, and seldom speaks to others.
d. "How dare you, a brand new employee, suggest we make these changes! We've always done it this way, and we will continue to do it this way! Those are the rules and they'll *not* be broken!"

9. Which of the following would be typical of an individual with obsessive-compulsive disorder?
   a. Receiving a paper cut, Linda yells, "Help me, quick! I'm bleeding! Somebody call 911!"
   b. Andrew becomes suspicious when John, who had an extra new year's calendar, left it on Andrew's desk as a gift.
   c. Fred works long hours in a solitary environment, lives alone, has no friends, and seldom speaks to others.
   • d. "How dare you, a brand new employee, suggest we make these changes! We've always done it this way, and we will continue to do it this way! Those are the rules and they'll *not* be broken!"

10. Which of the following would be typical of an individual with paranoid personality disorder?
   a. Receiving a paper cut, Linda yells, "Help me, quick! I'm bleeding! Somebody call 911!"
   • b. Andrew becomes suspicious when John, who had an extra new year's calendar, left it on Andrew's desk as a gift.
   c. Fred works long hours in a solitary environment, lives alone, has no friends, and seldom speaks to others.
   d. "How dare you, a brand new employee, suggest we make these changes! We've always done it this way, and we will continue to do it this way! Those are the rules and they'll *not* be broken!"

CHAPTER 21. CHILDREN AND ADOLESCENTS

CHAPTER FOCUS

The focus of this chapter is on psychiatric disorders usually first evident in infancy, childhood, or adolescence. Symptomatology and etiological implications are described. The role of the nurse in care of these clients is emphasized.

LEARNING OBJECTIVES

After reading this chapter, the student will be able to:
1. Identify psychiatric disorders usually first diagnosed in infancy, childhood, or adolescence.
2. Discuss etiological implications for mental retardation, autistic disorder, attention-deficit/hyperactivity disorder, conduct disorder, oppositional defiant disorder, Tourette's disorder, and separation anxiety disorder.
3. Identify symptomatology and use the information in the assessment of clients with the aforementioned disorders.
4. Identify nursing diagnoses common to clients with these disorders, and select appropriate nursing interventions for each.
5. Discuss relevant criteria for evaluating nursing care of clients with selected infant, childhood, and adolescent psychiatric disorders.
6. Describe treatment modalities relevant to selected disorders of infancy, childhood, and adolescence.

KEY TERMS

aggression
autistic disorder
temperament
impulsivity
negativism
clinging
palilalia
echolalia

CHAPTER OUTLINE/LECTURE NOTES

I. Introduction
   A. It is often difficult to determine if a child's behavior is indicative of emotional problems.
   B. The *DSM-IV-TR* suggests that an emotional problem exists if the behavioral manifestations:
      1. Are not age appropriate.

2. Deviate from cultural norms.
3. Create deficits or impairments in adaptive functioning.
II. Mental Retardation
   A. Defined by deficits in general intellectual functioning (as measured by intelligence quotient exams) and adaptive functioning (the ability to adapt to the requirements of daily living and the expectations of age and cultural group).
   B. Etiological implications
     1. Hereditary factors
       a. Implicated in approximately 5 percent of the cases. Includes:
         (1) Inborn errors of metabolism, such as Tay-Sachs disease, phenylketonuria, and hyperglycinemia.
         (2) Chromosomal disorders, such as Down's syndrome and Klinefelter's syndrome.
         (3) Single-gene abnormalities, such as tuberous sclerosis and neurofibromatosis.
     2. Early alterations in embryonic development
       a. Account for 30 percent of MR cases
       b. Damages may occur in response to:
         (1) Toxicity associated with maternal ingestion of alcohol or other drugs.
         (2) Maternal illnesses and infections during pregnancy.
         (3) Complications of pregnancy, such as toxemia and uncontrolled diabetes.
     3. Pregnancy and perinatal factors
       a. Account for approximately 10 percent of cases of MR
       b. Can be caused by:
         (1) Fetal malnutrition, viral, or other infections during pregnancy.
         (2) Trauma or complications of the birth process that result in deprivation of oxygen to the infant.
         (3) Premature birth.
     4. General medical conditions acquired in infancy or childhood
       a. Account for approximately 5 percent of cases of MR
       b. Can be caused by:
         (1) Infections, such as meningitis and encephalitis.
         (2) Poisonings, such as from insecticides, medications, or lead.
         (3) Physical traumas, such as head injuries, asphyxiation, and hyperpyrexia.
     5. Environmental influences and other mental disorders
       a. Accounts for approximately 20 percent of cases of MR
       b. May be attributed to:
         (1) Deprivation of nurturance and social, linguistic, and other stimulation.
         (2) Severe mental disorders, such as **autistic disorder.**
   C. Application of the nursing process
     1. Degree of severity of mental retardation is identified by level of intelligence quotient.
     2. Four levels have been delineated: mild, moderate, severe, and profound.

3. Nurses must access strengths as well as limitations in order to encourage the client to be as independent as possible.
4. It is important to include family members in the planning and implementation of care.
5. Family members should receive information regarding the scope of the condition, realistic expectations and client potentials, methods for modifying behavior as required, and community resources from whom they may seek assistance and support.
6. Evaluation of care given to the mentally retarded client should reflect positive behavioral change.

III. Autistic Disorder
   A. Characterized by a withdrawal of the child into the self and into a fantasy world of his or her own creation.
   B. The disorder is relatively rare and occurs 4 to 5 times more often in boys than in girls. Onset occurs prior to age 3 and in most cases runs a chronic course with symptoms persisting into adulthood.
   C. Etiological implications
      1. Social environment. Causative factors are thought to include parental rejection, child responses to deviant parental personality characteristics, family breakup, family stress, insufficient stimulation, and faulty communication patterns.
      2. Biological factors
         a. Genetics. Sibling and twin studies have revealed strong evidence that genetic factors play a significant role.
         b. Neurological factors. Early developmental problems have been implicated.
            (1) Postnatal neurological infections, congenital rubella, phenylketonuria, and fragile X syndrome
            (2) Various structural and functional abnormalities, including ventricular enlargement, left temporal abnormalities, increased glucose metabolism, and elevated blood serotonin level may also be involved.
   D. Application of the nursing process
      1. Background assessment data (symptomatology)
         a. Impairment in social interaction
         b. Impairment in communication and imaginative activity
         c. Restricted activities and interests
      2. Nursing intervention is aimed at protection of the child from self-directed violence, and improvement in social functioning, verbal communication, and personal identity.

VI. Attention-deficit/hyperactivity disorder (ADHD)
   A. Essential features include developmentally inappropriate degrees of inattention, impulsiveness, and hyperactivity.
   B. The disorder is further categorized into 3 subtypes:
      1. ADHD, Combined Type
      2. ADHD, Predominantly Inattentive Type
      3. ADHD, Predominantly Hyperactive-Impulsive Type

C. Etiological implications
   1. Biological influences
      a. Genetics. Frequency among family members has been noted.
      b. Biochemical theory. Implicates a deficit of dopamine and norepinephrine in the brain.
      c. Prenatal, perinatal, and postnatal factors
         (1) Prenatal factors include maternal smoking during pregnancy.
         (2) Perinatal factors include prematurity, signs of fetal distress, prolonged labor, and perinatal asphyxia.
         (3) Postnatal factors include cerebral palsy, epilepsy, and CNS trauma or infections.
   2. Environmental influences
      a. Environmental lead
      b. Diet factors, including food dyes and additives, and sugar
   3. Psychosocial influences
      a. Disorganized or chaotic environments
      b. Disruption in bonding during the first 3 years of life
      c. Family history of alcoholism, hysterical or sociopathic behaviors
      d. Parental history of hyperactivity
      e. Developmental learning disorders
D. Application of the nursing process
   1. Background assessment data (symptomatology)
      a. Highly distractible with extremely limited attention span
      b. Difficulty forming satisfactory interpersonal relationships
      c. Low frustration tolerance and outbursts of temper
      d. Excessive levels of activity, restlessness, and fidgeting
   2. Nursing intervention is aimed at protection from injury due to excessive hyperactivity, improvement in social interaction, self-esteem, and compliance with task expectations.
   3. Psychopharmacological intervention
      a. Drug of choice: CNS stimulants
      b. Examples: dextroamphetamine (Dexadrine), methylphenidate (Ritalin), dextroamphetamine/amphetamine composite (Adderall), and pemoline (Cylert)
      c. Effects on children with ADHD: increased attention span, control of hyperactive behavior, and improvement in learning ability
      d. Side effects: insomnia, anorexia, weight loss, tachycardia, and temporary decrease in rate of growth and development. Tolerance can occur. The drug should not be withdrawn abruptly.
      e. A drug "holiday" should be attempted periodically under direction of the physician to determine effectiveness of the medication and need for continuation.
V. Conduct Disorder

A. A repetitive and persistent pattern of behavior in which the basic rights of others or major age-appropriate societal norms or rules are violated. Two subtypes based on age at onset:
   1. Childhood-onset type: defined by the onset of at least one criterion characteristic of conduct disorder prior to age 10
   2. Adolescent-onset type: defined by the absence of any criteria characteristic of conduct disorder prior to age 10
B. Etiological implications
   1. Biological influences
      a. Genetics. Twin and non-twin sibling studies indicate a higher incidence among those who have family members with the disorder.
      b. **Temperament**. Children who are born with "difficult" temperaments were found to have a significantly higher degree of aggressive behavior later in life.
      c. Biochemical. Elevated levels of plasma testosterone have been correlated with aggressive behavior.
   2. Psychosocial influences
      a. Impaired social cognition. Rejection by peers may predispose to aggressive behavior.
      b. Family influences
         (1) The following family dynamics may contribute to the development of conduct disorder:
            (a) Parental rejection.
            (b) Inconsistent management with harsh discipline.
            (c) Early institutional living.
            (d) Frequent shifting of parental figures.
            (e) Large family size.
            (f) Absent father.
            (g) Parents with antisocial personality disorder or alcohol dependence.
            (h) Association with a delinquent subgroup.
            (i) Marital conflict and divorce.
            (j) Inadequate communication patterns.
            (k) Parental permissiveness.
C. Application of the nursing process
   1. Background assessment data (symptomatology)
      a. Physical **aggression** in the violation of the rights of others
      b. Use of drugs and alcohol
      c. Sexual permissiveness
      d. Use of projection as a defense mechanism
      e. Low self-esteem manifested by "tough-guy" image
      f. Inability to control anger
      g. Low academic achievement
   2. Nursing intervention is aimed at protection of others from client's physical aggression; improvement in social interaction and self-esteem; and acceptance of responsibility for own behavior.

VI. Oppositional Defiant Disorder (ODD)
  A. Characterized by a pattern of negativistic, defiant, disobedient, and hostile behavior toward authority figures that occurs more frequently than is typically observed in individuals of comparable age and developmental level, and interferes with social, academic, or occupational functioning.
  B. Etiological implications
    1. Biological influences. Role not established.
    2. Family influences. If power and control are issues for parents, or if they exercise authority for their own needs, a power struggle can be established between the parents and the child that sets the stage for the development of ODD.
  C. Application of the nursing process
    1. Background assessment data (symptomatology)
      a. Symptoms include passive-aggression, exhibited by obstinacy, procrastination, disobedience, carelessness, **negativism**, dawdling, provocation, resistance to change, violation of minor rules, blocking out communications from others, and resistance to authority.
      b. Other symptoms may include enuresis, encopresis, elective mutism, running away, school avoidance, school underachievement, eating and sleeping problems, temper tantrums, fighting, and argumentativeness.
      c. Interpersonal relationships are impaired and school performance is often unsatisfactory.
    2. Nursing intervention is aimed at compliance with therapy, acceptance of responsibility for own behavior, increase in self-esteem, and improvement in social interaction.
VII. Tourette's Disorder
  A. The essential feature is the presence of multiple motor tics and one or more vocal tics.
  B. Onset of the disorder is before age 18 and is more common in boys than in girls.
  C. Etiological implications
    1. Biological factors
      a. Genetics. Twin studies suggest an inheritable component. The familial predisposition to tic disorders appears to be governed by a single gene with autosomal dominant transmission.
      b. Biochemical factors. Abnormalities in levels of dopamine, serotonin, dynorphin, gamma-aminobutyric acid, acetylcholine, and norepinephrine have been associated with Tourette's disorder.
      c. Structural factors. Brain studies in Tourette's disorder have found enlargement in the caudate nucleus and decreased cerebral blood flow in the left ventricular nucleus.
    2. Environmental factors
      a. Increased prenatal complications and lower birth weight
      b. Greater emotional stress during pregnancy and more nausea and vomiting during the first trimester of pregnancy have been noted in the mothers of these children.

D. Application of the nursing process
   1. Background assessment data (symptomatology)
      a. Simple motor tics include eye blinking, neck jerking, shoulder shrugging, facial grimacing, and coughing.
      b. Complex motor tics include touching, squatting, hopping, skipping, deep knee bends, retracing steps, and twirling when walking.
      c. Vocal tics include words or sounds such as clicks, grunts, yelps, barks, sniffs, snorts, coughs, and rarely, the uttering of obscenities.
      d. Vocal tics may also include repeating one's own sounds or words (called **palilalia**), or repeating the words of others (called **echolalia**).
   2. Nursing intervention is aimed at protection of the client and others, improvement in social interaction, and improvement in self-esteem.
   3. Pharmacological intervention with Tourette's disorder is most effective when it is combined with other forms of therapy, such as education and supportive intervention, individual counseling or psychotherapy, and family therapy. The most common medications used are:
      a. Haloperidol (Haldol). Because of the severe side effects, this medication should be reserved for children with severe symptoms or with symptoms that impede their ability to function in school, socially, or within their family setting.
      b. Pimozide (Orap). Similar in response rate and side effect profile to haloperidol. Used only with severe cases. Not recommended for children under age 12.
      c. Clonidine (Catapres). Sometimes used as drug of first choice because of few side effects. Results of studies on the efficacy of clonidine in the treatment of Tourette's disorder have been mixed.
VIII. Separation Anxiety Disorder
   A. Essential feature of this disorder is excessive anxiety concerning separation from the home or from those to whom the person is attached.
   B. Etiological implications
      1. Biological influences
         a. Genetics. Studies show that a greater number of children with relatives who manifest anxiety problems develop anxiety disorders themselves than do children with no such family patterns.
         b. Temperament. It is believed that certain individuals inherit a "disposition" toward developing anxiety disorders.
      2. Environmental influences
         a. Stressful life events. It is thought that children who are already predisposed to developing anxiety disorders may be affected significantly by stressful life events.
      3. Family influences
         a. Possible over-attachment to the mother
         b. Separation conflicts between parent and child
         c. Families that are very close-knit
         d. Overprotection by parents

    e.   Transfer of fears and anxieties from parents to child through role modeling

C. Application of the nursing process

    1. Background assessment data (symptomatology)

        a. Onset of separation anxiety disorder may occur as early as preschool age, rarely as late as adolescence.

        b. Child has difficulty separating from mother

        c. Separation results in tantrums, crying, screaming, complaints of physical problems, and "**clinging**" behaviors.

        d. School reluctance or refusal

        e. Fear of sleeping away from home

        f. Fear of harm to self or attachment figure

        g. Nightmares may occur

        h. Phobias and depressed mood are not uncommon

    2. Nursing intervention is aimed at maintaining anxiety at moderate level or below; improvement in social interaction; and development of adaptive coping strategies that prevent maladaptive symptoms of anxiety in response to separation from attachment figure.

IX. Summary

X. Critical Thinking Exercise

XI. Review Questions

ANSWERS TO CRITICAL THINKING EXERCISE:

1. Assessment data: behavior unmanageable, yells, interrupts, is physically aggressive, can't sit still, jumps from topic to topic, no insight into his own behavior, refusing to cooperate

2. Risk for other-directed violence

3. Noncompliance and defensive coping

CASE STUDIES FOR USE WITH STUDENT LEARNING

Case Study No. 1: Autistic Disorder *

Seth, age 3, is the third child (and only boy) of Tom and Sue. He has been referred to a psychiatrist by their family physician at the request of the parents. Sue reports that she had a very difficult delivery of Seth, and he had needed oxygen at birth. Tom and Sue report that, from the very beginning, Seth has been "different" from their other children who have always enjoyed social interaction. Seth has tended to be aloof with a lack of response to social contact. When left with a baby sitter, he often screams much of the time. His speech is limited and often confusing. For example, he often echos words and phrases he hears or has heard in the past. He may state, "Do you want to eat?" to indicate that he is hungry. His words are monotonistic and carry little, if any, inflection. He is fascinated by two things: objects that turn and music. He loves to listen to music and often dances in circles when listening. He has a favorite spinning top that he likes to carry around with him at all times. He is an expert at putting together jigsaw puzzles. He also likes to distribute kitchen utensils (particularly those with spinning parts) to various places around the house, and retrieval by Mom for their original use may precipitate temper tantrums lasting an hour or more, with screaming, kicking, and biting himself or others. Restoration of the status quo, playing his favorite music, or a long car ride is often the only way to interrupt these tantrums. The psychiatrist admits Seth to the child psychatric unit where he is given a diagnosis of Autistic Disorder. Design a nursing plan of care for Seth.

_____

* Adapted from: Spitzer, R.L. et al. (1994). *DSM-IV Case Book*. Washington, D.C., American Psychiatric Press, Inc.

Case Study No. 2: Attention-Deficit/Hyperactivity Disorder*

Frankie is a 9-year-old boy who, according to his teacher, is constantly "into everything." He keeps the class in an uproar, and has been suspended from school three times this year, most recently for swinging from a light fixture. He wanders around the classroom talking to all the children, so that not only does Frankie not accomplish *his* work, the other students cannot complete *theirs* either. Frankie's mother reports that Frankie's behavior has been difficult since he was a toddler, when he became unbearably restless and demanding. He slept very little and "got into everything." When he was 4 years old, he was rejected by a preschool because of his difficult behavior. He has few friends because he is unable to participate in fair play. He is unable to watch TV or participate in games that require quiet concentration. His activities at home essentially include riding his bike or playing outdoors with his dog. His room stays messy and he is destructive of his possessions. The psychiatrist admits Frankie to the child psychiatric unit with a diagnosis of ADHD. He orders initiation of therapy with methylphenidate (Ritalin). Design a nursing plan of care for Frankie.

_____

*Adapted from: Spitzer, R.J. et at. (1994). *DSM-IV Case Book*. Washington, D.C.: American Psychiatric Press, Inc.

LEARNING ACTIVITY

DISORDERS OF INFANCY, CHILDHOOD, OR ADOLESCENCE

Match the disorders listed on the left to the behaviors associated with each on the right.

_____ 1. Mild Mental Retardation

a. No capacity for independent functioning. IQ below 20.

_____ 2. Autistic Disorder

b. Violates the rights of others and societal norms and rules. Physical aggression and inability to control anger.

_____ 3. Moderate Mental Retardation

c. Negativistic and defiant behavior, including obstinacy, procrastination, disobedience, resistance to change and authority.

_____ 4. Conduct Disorder

d. May be trained in elementary hygiene skills. Requires complete supervision. IQ 20-34.

_____ 5. Severe Mental Retardation

e. Withdrawal of the child into the self and into a fantasy world of his or her own creation.

_____ 6. Separation Anxiety Disorder

f. Developmentally inappropriate degrees of inattention, impulsiveness, and hyperactivity.

_____ 7. Attention-Deficit/Hyperactivity Disorder

g. Screams and throws temper tantrums at anticipated separation from mother. Fear of harm to self or mother.

_____ 8. Tourette's Disorder

h. Capable of developing social skills and independent living, with assistance. IQ 50-70.

_____ 9. Oppositional Defiant Disorder	i. Presence of multiple motor tics and one or more vocal tics.
_____10. Profound Mental Retardation	j. Capable of academic skill to second grade level. IQ 35-49.

TEST QUESTIONS

1. Glenda, diagnosed as mentally retarded, recently had IQ testing, and scored 47. Her parents have called a local agency that serves the developmentally disabled, and asked for advice regarding Glenda's potential. Which of the following statements from the nurse who counsels them is the *best* estimate of Glenda's eventual level of development?
   a. "Glenda may develop minimal verbal skills."
   - b. "Glenda may be able to work at an unskilled job."
   c. "Glenda may eventually function at about a sixth grade level."
   d. "Glenda will require constant supervision and care."

2. The nurse counselor develops a long-term plan for Glenda, based on nursing diagnoses appropriate to her potential level of function. Which of the following nursing diagnoses is *most appropriate* for Glenda?
   - a. Self-care deficit related to lack of maturity
   b. Impaired social interaction related to speech difficulties
   c. Risk for injury related to aggressive behavior
   d. Altered growth and development related to inadequate environmental stimulation

3. Tommy, age 9, has been diagnosed with autistic disorder. The cause of this disorder is thought to be:
   a. Refrigerator parents.
   b. Fragile X syndrome.
   c. Increased glucose metabolism.
   - d. The cause is unknown.

4. A psychiatric nurse frequently visits Tommy and his parents and brother Ronnie, age 3. Which of the following behaviors would the nurse regard as age-appropriate and *not* indicative of autistic disorder?
   a. Intense fascination with fans

- b. Parallel play
  - c. Lack of eye contact
  - d. Drinking large quantities of fluid

5. Tommy's mother tells the psychiatric nurse that Ronnie is in constant motion and is unable to sit long enough to listen to a story or even to watch TV. She asks the nurse if she thinks he could be "hyperactive." The nurse's *best* response is:
   - a. "I wouldn't worry about it."
   - b. "It's certainly possible."
   - c. "It's hard to tell with a 3-year-old."
   - d. "Why would you think that?"

6. Which of the following factors would prompt the nurse to continue to evaluate Ronnie for ADHD?
   - a. Ronnie's father smokes.
   - b. Ronnie was born 7 weeks prematurely.
   - c. Ronnie develops hives when he eats foods with red food coloring added.
   - d. Ronnie has a cousin on his father's side who has ADHD.

7. Calming effects on hyperactive children have been found to occur with the administration of which of the following classifications of medications?
   - a. CNS stimulants
   - b. CNS depressants
   - c. NSAIDs
   - d. Antimanic drugs, such as lithium

8. A potential side effect from prolonged use of methylphenidate (Ritalin) is which of the following?
   - a. Psychosis
   - b. Decreased intelligence
   - c. Dry mouth and sore throat
   - d. Decrease in rate of growth and development

9. The *primary* nursing intervention in working with a child with a conduct disorder is to:
   - a. Plan activities that provide opportunities for success.
   - b. Give the child unconditional acceptance for good behaviors that occur.
   - c. Recognize behaviors that precede the onset of aggression and intervene before violence occurs.
   - d. Provide immediate positive feedback for acceptable and unacceptable

behaviors.

10. Which of the following classes of medications is effective in the treatment of Tourette's Disorder?
    - • a. Neuroleptics
      b. Antimanics
      c. Tricyclic antidepressants
      d. Monoamine oxidase inhibitors

11. In providing care for the adolescent with an overanxious disorder, the *primary* goal of the nurse is:
    a. To set very strict limits on what behavior can be tolerated.
    b. To make the adolescent aware of the outcome of his or her desire to excel.
    - • c. To establish an atmosphere of calm trust and unconditional acceptance.
      d. To accept all "nervous habit" behavior and extinguish somatic symptoms.

12. The essential feature that distinguishes Oppositional Defiant Disorder from other disorders is:
    a. Gender ratio.
    - • b. Passive-aggressiveness.
      c. Violence toward others.
      d. The role of genetic predisposition.

CHAPTER 22. VICTIMS OF ABUSE OR NEGLECT

CHAPTER FOCUS

The focus of this chapter is on nursing care of clients experiencing problems related to abuse or neglect. Etiological implications and symptomatology are explored, and nursing care is presented in the context of the six steps of the nursing process. Various treatment modalities are also discussed.

LEARNING OBJECTIVES

After reading this chapter, the student will be able to:
1. Discuss historical perspectives associated with spouse abuse, child abuse, and sexual assault.
2. Describe epidemiological statistics associated with spouse abuse, child abuse, and sexual assault.
3. Discuss characteristics of victims and victimizers.
4. Identify etiological implications for abusive behaviors.
5. Describe physical and psychological effects on the victim of spouse abuse, child abuse, and sexual assault.
6. Identify nursing diagnoses, goals of care, and appropriate nursing interventions for care of victims of spouse abuse, child abuse, and sexual assault.
7. Evaluate nursing care of victims of spouse abuse, child abuse, and sexual assault.
8. Discuss various modalities relevant to treatment of victims of abuse.

KEY TERMS

battering	rape
child sexual abuse	date rape
emotional injury	marital rape
emotional neglect	statutory rape
physical neglect	incest
safe house or shelter	compounded rape reaction
controlled response pattern	expressed response pattern
silent rape reaction	sexual exploitation of a child
	cycle of battering

CHAPTER OUTLINE/LECTURE NOTES

I. Introduction
   A. *Abuse* is the maltreatment of one person by another.
   B. **Battering** is the single most common cause of injury to women.
   C. An increase in the incidence of child abuse has been documented.
II. Historical Perspectives

A. Spouse and child abuse arrived in the United States with the Puritans. Women and children were viewed as personal property of men.

B. The notion of women as subordinate and subservient to men, as well as that of "spare the rod and spoil the child," was supported by the *Bible*.

C. Not until the second half of the twentieth century has legal protection been available for victims of abuse.

III. Etiological Implications

A. Biological theories

1. Neurophysiological influences. Areas of the brain that have been implicated in both the facilitation and inhibition of aggressive impulses include the temporal lobe, the limbic system, and the amygdaloid nucleus.

2. Biochemical influences. Certain neurotransmitters, including norepinephrine, serotonin, and dopamine, have been implicated in the regulation of aggressive impulses.

3. Genetic influences. A possible hereditary factor may be involved. The genetic karyotype XYY has also been implicated.

4. Disorders of the brain. Aggressive and violent behavior has been correlated with organic brain syndromes, brain tumors, brain trauma, encephalitis, and temporal lobe epilepsy.

B. Psychological theories

1. Psychodynamic theory. Unmet needs for satisfaction and security result in an underdeveloped ego and a weak superego. Aggression and violence supply the individual with a dose of power and prestige that boosts the self-image and validates a significance to his or her life that is lacking.

2. Learning theory. Children learn to behave by imitating their role models. Individuals who were abused as children or whose parents disciplined with physical punishment are more likely to behave in an abusive manner as adults.

C. Sociocultural theories

1. Societal influences. Aggressive behavior is primarily a product of one's culture and social structure. The American culture was founded on a general acceptance of violence as a means of solving problems.

2. Societal influences also contribute to violence when individuals realize that their needs and desires are not being met relative to other persons.

IV. Application of the nursing process: background assessment data

A. Spouse abuse

1. *Spouse abuse* has been defined as "the mistreatment or misuse of one spouse by the other. It can range from shoving and pushing to choking and severe battering, involving broken limbs, broken ribs, internal bleeding, and brain damage."

2. Profile of the victim. Battered women represent all age, racial, religious, cultural, educational, and socioeconomic groups. They often have low self-esteem. They may be without adequate support systems. Many grew up in abusive homes.

3. Profile of the victimizer. Men who batter are generally characterized as persons with low self-esteem, pathologically jealous, presenting a "dual

personality," exhibiting limited coping ability and severe stress reactions. The spouse is viewed as a personal possession.

4. The **cycle of battering**. Three distinct phases:
   a. Phase I. Tension-building phase
   b. Phase II. Acute battering incident
   c. Phase III. Calm, loving, respite (honeymoon) phase
5. Why does she stay? The most frequent response to this question is that they fear for their life or the lives of their children. Other reasons given include a lack of support network for leaving, religious beliefs, and a lack of financial independence to support herself and her children.

B. Child abuse
   1. Physical injury. Any nonaccidental physical injury, caused by the parent or caregiver.
      a. Physical signs
      b. Behavioral signs
   2. **Emotional injury.** A pattern of behavior on the part of the parent or caretaker that results in serious impairment of the child's social, emotional, or intellectual functioning.
      a. Behavioral indicators
   3. Neglect
      a. **Physical neglect.** Includes refusal of or delay in seeking health care, abandonment, expulsion from the home or refusal to allow a runaway to return home, and inadequate supervision
         (1) Physical and behavioral indicators
      b. **Emotional Neglect.** Refers to a chronic failure by the parent or caretaker to provide the child with the hope, love, and support necessary for the development of a sound, healthy personality
         (1) Behavioral indicators
   4. Sexual abuse of a child
      a. **Sexual exploitation of a child**. When a child is induced or coerced into engaging in sexually explicit conduct for the purpose of promoting any performance
      b. Sexual abuse. When a child is being used for the sexual pleasure of an adult (parent or caretaker) or any other person
      c. **Incest**. The occurrence of sexual contacts or interaction between, or sexual exploitation of, close relatives, or between participants who are related to each other by a kinship bond that is regarded as a prohibition to sexual relations (for example, caretakers, stepparents, stepsiblings)
      d. Indicators of sexual abuse
         (1) Physical indicators
         (2) Behavioral indicators
   5. Characteristics of the abuser
      a. Parents who abuse their children were likely abused as children themselves.

b. Experiencing a stressful life situation (for example, unemployment, poverty)

c. Having few, if any, support systems

d. Lacking understanding of child development or care needs

e. Lacking adaptive coping strategies; angers easily; has difficulty trusting others

f. Expecting the child to be perfect; may exaggerate any mild difference the child manifests from the "usual"

6. The incestual relationship

a. Often there is an impaired spousal relationship.

b. Father is often domineering, impulsive, and physically abusing.

c. Mother is commonly passive, submissive, and denigrates her role of wife and mother. She is often aware of, or at least suspects, the incestuous relationship, but uses denial or keeps quiet out of fear of being abused by her husband.

7. The adult survivor of incest

a. Common characteristics:

(1) A fundamental lack of trust that arises out of an unsatisfactory parent-child relationship.

(2) Low self-esteem and a poor sense of identity.

(3) Absence of pleasure with sexual activity.

(4) Promiscuity.

C. Sexual assault

1. **Rape** is an act of aggression, not one of passion. It is identified by the use of force and executed "against the person's will."

a. **Date rape**. Applied to sexual assault in which the rapist is known to the victim

b. **Marital rape**. Sexual violence directed at a marital partner against that person's will

c. **Statutory rape**. Unlawful intercourse between a man older than 16 years of age and a woman under the age of consent

2. Profile of the victimizer .

a. The mother of the rapist has been described as "seductive but rejecting" toward her child. She is overbearing, with seductive undertones, but is quick to withdraw her "love" and attention when he goes against her wishes. Her dominance over her son often continues into his adult life.

b. Many rapists report growing up in abusive homes. Even when the abuse was discharged by the father, the rapist's anger is directed toward the mother for not providing adequate protection from the father's abuse.

c. More recent feminist theories suggest that the rapist displaces anger on the rape victim because he cannot directly express it toward other men.

3. The victim

a. Rape can occur at any age. The highest risk group appears to be between 16 and 24 years.

    b. Most victims are single women, and the attack often occurs near their own neighborhood.

    c. When the attack is a "stranger rape," victims are not chosen for any reason having to do with their appearance or behavior, but simply because they happened to be in that place at that particular time.

    d. The presence of a weapon (real or perceived) appears to be the principal measure of the degree to which a woman resists her attacker.

    e. Victim responses:

        (1) **Expressed response pattern**—the victim expresses feelings of fear, anger, and anxiety through such behaviors as crying, sobbing, smiling, restlessness, and tension.

        (2) **Controlled response pattern**—feelings of the victim are masked or hidden, and a calm, composed, or subdued affect is seen.

        (3) **Compounded rape reaction**—additional symptoms such as depression and suicide, substance abuse, and even psychotic behaviors may be noted in the victim.

        (4) **Silent rape reaction**—the victim tells no one about the assault. Anxiety is suppressed, and the emotional burden may become overwhelming.

V. Diagnoses/Outcome Identification

    A. Nursing diagnoses for the client who has been abused may include:

      1. Rape-trauma syndrome.

      2. Powerlessness.

      3. Altered growth and development.

    B. Outcome criteria are identified for measuring the effectiveness of nursing care.

VI. Planning/Implementation

    A. Nursing intervention for the victim of abuse or neglect is to provide shelter and promote reassurance of his or her safety.

    B. Other nursing concerns include:

      1. Tending to physical injuries.

      2. Staying with the client to provide security.

      3. Assisting the client to recognize options.

      4. Promoting trust.

      5. Reporting to authorities when there is "reason to suspect" child abuse or neglect.

VII. Evaluation is based on accomplishment of previously established outcome criteria.

VIII. Treatment Modalities

    A. Crisis intervention

    B. **Safe house or shelter**

    C. Family therapy

IX. Summary

X. Critical Thinking Exercise

XI. Review Questions

ANSWERS TO CRITICAL THINKING EXERCISE

1. "He doesn't act this way because of anything you do."
2. Powerlessness related to cycle of battering
3. The nurse must help Lisa understand that alternatives to her current situation do exist, and it is her decision to choose one of the alternatives or return to her current living situation. Either way, she will be supported in her decision.

CASE STUDY FOR USE WITH STUDENT LEARNING

Case Study: Physical Neglect of a Child

Amy, age 5, started kindergarten this year. Her teacher noticed that she seems to spend a lot of time alone, standing on the sidelines during recess watching the other children play, but not entering into the interaction. She comes to school somewhat unkempt with a noticeable body odor about her. She participates in the free school lunch program, and often gulps her food, appearing ravenous when the food is presented. As the weather turns cold, the teacher notices that Amy is coming to school without a coat. When questioned, she states, "I don't have a coat." The teacher reports Amy's case to the DHS and a home health nurse is sent to Amy's home to investigate. At Amy's home the nurse finds a teenager who identifies herself as Amy's sister, Carol. She is caring for three other children: an 8-year-old boy and a 3-year-old girl, whom she identifies as her siblings, and a 6-month-old girl, whom she identifies as her own child. There is no adult in the home. Carol tells the nurse that she is 16 years old and has full charge of these children most of the time. Carol's mother lives with her boyfriend most of the time, but comes to the house occasionally to bring a few groceries. Carol tells the nurse that she is worried because the electric company has threatened to turn off the electricity for lack of payment and because there has been no food in the house for 2 days. She says she has talked to her mother several times, but her mother just responds that she doesn't have any money right now, and they must do the best that they can. DHS places all the children in foster care and tells the mother that she must undergo therapy in order to justify return of the children to her care. Devise a plan of care that the home health nurse might use to assist the mother in this effort.

LEARNING ACTIVITY

BEHAVIORS OF ABUSE OR NEGLECT

Match the terms on the right to the situations they describe on the left.

_____ 1. John likes to brag of his sexual conquests to his friends.   a. Physical injury
When Alice rejected his sexual advances on their first date,
he became angry and forced intercourse with her.

_____ 2. Alice tells no one about the encounter with John. She   b. Compounded rape
suppresses her anxiety and tries to pretend it didn't happen.   reaction

_____ 3. Harry is 28 years old. He is very flattered when 15-year-old   c. Spouse abuse
Lisa pays attention to him at a party. After the party, he takes
her to his home, where she agrees to have sex with him.

_____ 4. At 9 P.M., Jack comes home intoxicated from the bar where he had   d. Date rape
gone after work with his friends. When he finds his dinner cold, he
slaps his wife across the face, knocks her down, and kicks her.

_____ 5. Jack pulls his wife to their bed, and against her protests,   e. Expressed response
forces intercourse with her, yelling, "You can't say no to me!   pattern
You're my wife!"

_____ 6. Janie is 6 years old. Her father left home a year ago and has never returned. Her mother frequently says to Janie, "See what you did?! If you had been a better little girl, Daddy wouldn't have left us!"

f. Incest

_____ 7. Janie attempts to establish a relationship with her mother, but whenever Janie approaches her mother for interaction, her mother yells, "Get away from me! I don't want to have anything to do with bad little girls!"

g. Marital rape

_____ 8. Janie has open sores on her buttocks. She tells the babysitter, "My mommy made them with her cigarette."

h. Statutory rape

_____ 9. Janie comes to school in the snow without a coat. When asked where her coat is, Janie replies, "I don't have one."

i. Silent rape reaction

_____ 10. Scarlet is 15 years old. She is sent to the school nurse by her homeroom teacher. She is obviously having symptoms of a panic attack. Upon becoming calmer, Scarlet explains to the nurse that Frank just asked her for her first date. With much encouragement, the nurse learns that Scarlet's father has been coming into her bed at night for 5 years now. At first he just touched and fondled her, but last year he began having intercourse with her.

j. Emotional injury

_____ 11. After being raped by a man in the deserted laundry room of her apartment building, Carol is taken to the hospital by her roommate. Carol is sobbing and yelling, "He had no right to do that to me!" She is tense, and is fearful of any man who comes near her.

k. Emotional neglect

_____ 12. Carol's physical wounds heal, but in subsequent weeks, she becomes increasingly fearful. She is overcome with despair and talks of taking her life. She drinks a great deal of alcohol to help her get through each day.

l. Physical neglect

TEST QUESTIONS

Situation: Roberta is a 43-year-old married woman who has called in sick to work for 3 days. When she finally returns to work, her makeup cannot conceal bruises on her face. A coworker who is a good friend mentions the bruises, and says they look like the bruises she used to have after being beaten by her former husband. Roberta says, "It was an accident. He just had a terrible day at work. He's being so kind and gentle now. Yesterday he brought me flowers. He says he's going to get a new job, so it won't ever happen again."

1. Which phase of the cycle of battering does Roberta's response represent?
    a. Phase I. The Tension-Building Phase
    b. Phase II. The Acute Battering Incident
    • c. Phase III. The Honeymoon Phase
    d. Phase IV. The Resolution Phase

2. Roberta's coworker recommends that she seek assistance from her Employee Assistance Program. Roberta refuses because she believes her husband has reformed. What is the *best* alternative suggestion her coworker can make at this point?
    a. Buy a gun.
    b. File for divorce
    c. Press charges of assault and battery.
 • d. Carry the number of the safe house for battered women.

Situation: Katie is a 9-year-old third grader. Her teacher, Mrs. Small, notices that Katie has had an open lesion on her left arm for a week. The lesion appears to have become infected, which is easy to see because Mrs. Small has never seen it covered with a bandage. Katie is often absent from school, and seems apathetic and tired when she attends. Other children in the classroom avoid her, and Mrs. Small has overheard them talking about Katie stealing food from them at lunchtime.

3. Mrs. Small's observations are indications of which of the following?
 • a. Physical neglect
    b. Emotional injury
    c. Physical abuse
    d. Sexual abuse

Situation: Teresa, an unmarried 37-year-old woman, has recently been referred from her family physician to the psychiatrist with the complaint of "anxiety attacks." These attacks occur in the evening before bedtime, and Teresa has also been experiencing insomnia. When she does get to sleep, she often has nightmares. She tells the psychiatrist that her father has recently been diagnosed with an inoperable brain tumor.

4. What might the psychiatrist suspect after making his initial assessment of Teresa?
    a. Possible depressive disorder.
 • b. Possible history of childhood incest
    c. Possible anticipatory grieving
    d. Possible history of childhood physical abuse

Situation: The police escort Zoe, a 29-year-old, married stock market analyst, to the emergency department (ED) of an inner-city hospital. She is sobbing, her clothing is torn and she has superficial cuts on her neck and chest. She was leaving her office after working late and was accosted from behind as she bent to unlock her car, which was parked at the periphery of the parking lot. Her assailant raped her and stole her purse and her car. She walked to a nearby telephone, dialed 911, and a police car was dispatched to assist her. Upon arrival at the ED, the triage nurse immediately calls a member of the Sexual Assault Crisis Team, who arrives within 20 minutes and remains with Zoe throughout her stay in the ED.

5. What is the most therapeutic thing for the nurse to say to Zoe when she arrives at the ED?
   - • a. "You are safe now."
   - b. "I'll call your husband."
   - c. "The police will want to interview you."
   - d. "We'll have to take photographs of those wounds."

6. Zoe is crying, pacing, and cursing her attacker. Which behavioral defense do these manifestations represent?
   - a. Controlled response pattern
   - b. Compounded rape reaction
   - • c. Expressed response pattern
   - d. Silent rape reaction

General questions related to abuse and neglect:

7. Sally was raped by a man with whom she had been on a "blind" date. She did not report the assault, but in the months that followed, she became very depressed, began to drink a great deal, and thought about taking her own life. Which emotional defense response do these behavioral manifestations represent?
   - a. Expressed response pattern
   - b. Controlled response pattern
   - c. Silent rape reaction
   - • d. Compounded rape reaction

8. Lucy, age 7, is crying at school. She tells the nurse that her Mommy doesn't love her. When the nurse asks her to explain, Lucy says, "Mommy said Daddy left us because I was a bad girl, and she doesn't love bad girls." The nurse assesses this behavior on the part of Lucy's mother as possible:
   - • a. Emotional injury
   - b. Physical abuse
   - c. Physical neglect
   - d. Emotional neglect

9. Marie and her husband appear at the emergency department of a large hospital. Marie has a swollen, black eye and various cuts and bruises on her face, some of which are

bleeding. Marie's husband tells the triage nurse that Marie tripped and fell off their back porch. Marie is quiet and does not add to the report. The nurse does not believe that the injuries are consistent with the husband's report of the accident. How should the nurse proceed with this case?

    a. Tell Marie that she doesn't believe her husband's story.
    b. Ask Marie why she isn't talking.
- c. Take Marie to another room by herself to interview her.
    d. Report the incident to the police.

10. A woman who experiences spouse abuse states, "I know he loves me. He wouldn't beat me, except that he drinks a lot because he's under so much stress at work." This woman is using which defense mechanism?

    a. Suppression
    b. Repression
    c. Denial
- d. Rationalization

CHAPTER 23. THE AGING INDIVIDUAL

CHAPTER FOCUS

The focus of this chapter is on nursing care of the aging individual. Various theories of aging and symptomatology associated with the normal aging process are presented. Special concerns of the elderly are discussed. Nursing care is described in the context of the six steps of the nursing process.

LEARNING OBJECTIVES

After reading this chapter, the student will be able to:
1. Discuss societal perspectives on aging.
2. Describe an epidemiological profile of aging in the United States.
3. Discuss various theories of aging.
4. Describe aspects of the normal aging process, including:
    a. Biological.
    b. Psychological.
    c. Sociocultural.
    d. Sexual.
5. Discuss retirement as a special concern to the aging individual.
6. Explain personal and sociological perspectives of long-term care of the aging individual.
7. Describe the problem of elder abuse as it exists in today's society.
8. Discuss the implications of the increasing number of suicides among the elderly population.
9. Apply the steps of the nursing process to the care of aging individuals.

KEY TERMS

attachment
bereavement overload
disengagement
geriatrics
gerontology
geropsychiatry
"granny-bashing"
"granny-dumping"

long-term memory
short-term memory
reminiscence therapy
menopause
osteoporosis
Medicare
Medicaid

CHAPTER OUTLINE/LECTURE NOTES

I. Introduction
    A. Growing old is not popular in the youth-oriented American culture.

B. Sixty-six million "baby boomers" will reach their 65th birthdays by the year 2030, placing more emphasis on the needs of an aging population.

II. How Old is *Old*?

A. Our prehistoric ancestors probably had a life span of 40 years, with an average life span of 18 years.

B. By 1985, the average life expectancy at birth was 71.2 years for men and 78.2 for women.

C. Myths and stereotypes affect the way in which elderly people are treated in our culture.

D. Whether one is considered "old" must be self-determined, based on variables such as attitude, mental health, physical health, and degree of independence.

III. Epidemiological Statistics

A. Population

1. In 1998, Americans 65 years of age or older numbered 34.4 million, representing 12.7 percent of the population.

2. By 2030, this number is projected at 70 million, or 20 percent of the population.

B. Marital status

1. In 1998, 75 percent of men and 43 percent of women ages 65 or over were married.

2. There were four times as many widows as widowers.

C. Living arrangements: The majority of individuals ages 65 or over live alone, with a spouse, or with relatives.

D. Economic status: About 3.4 million persons age 65 or over were below the poverty level in 1998.

E. Employment: Individuals age 65 or over constituted 2.8 percent of the U.S. labor force in 1998.

F. Health status

1. The number of days in which usual activities are restricted because of illness or injury increases with age.

2. Emotional and mental illnesses also increase over the life cycle.

IV. Theories of Aging

A. Biological theories

1. The exhaustion theory

2. The accumulation theory

3. The biological programming theory

4. The error theory

5. The cross-linkage or eversion theory

6. The immunological theory

7. The "aging clock" theory

8. The free radical theory

B. Psychosocial theories

1. The activity theory of aging

2. Continuity theory

C. Personality theories

1. Mature men
2. Rocking chair
3. Armored men
4. Angry men
5. Self-haters

V. The Normal Aging Process
   A. Biological aspects of aging. Changes are observed in:
      1. Skin.
      2. Cardiovascular system.
      3. Respiratory system.
      4. Musculoskeletal system.
      5. Gastrointestinal system.
      6. Endocrine system.
      7. Genitourinary system.
      8. Immune system.
      9. Nervous system.
      10. Sensory systems.
   B. Psychological aspects of aging
      1. Memory functioning
      2. Intellectual functioning
      3. Learning ability.
      4. Adaptation to the tasks of aging
         a. Loss and grief
         b. **Attachment** and **disengagement**
         c. Maintenance of self-identity
         d. Dealing with death
         e. Psychiatric disorders in later life
   C. Sociocultural aspects of aging
      1. The elderly in virtually all cultures share some basic needs and interests:
         a. To live as long as possible or at least until life's satisfactions no longer compensate for its privations.
         b. To get some release from the necessity of wearisome exertion at humdrum tasks and to have protection from too great exposure to physical hazards.
         c. To safeguard or even strengthen any prerogatives acquired in midlife, such as skills, possessions, rights, authority, and prestige.
         d. To remain active participants in the affairs of life in either operational or supervisory roles, any sharing in group interests being preferred to idleness and indifference.
         e. To withdraw from life when necessity requires it, as timely, honorably, and comfortably as possible.
      2. In some cultures, the aged are the most powerful, the most engaged, and the most respected members of the society. This has not been the case in the American culture.
   D. Sexual aspects of aging

1. Americans have grown up in a society that has liberated sexual expression for all other age groups, but still retains certain Victorian standards regarding sexual expression by the elderly.
2. Cultural stereotypes play a large part in the misperception many people hold regarding sexuality of the aged.
3. Physical changes associated with sexuality
   a. Changes in the female
   b. Changes in the male
4. Sexual behavior in the elderly

VI. Special Concerns of the Elderly Population
   A. Retirement
      1. Social implications
      2. Economic implications
   B. Long-term care
      1. Potential need for services are predicted by the following factors:
         a. Age. The 65+ population is often viewed as one of the important long-term-care target groups.
         b. Health. The requirement for ongoing assistance from another human being is a consideration.
         c. Mental health status. Symptoms that would render the individual incapable of meeting the demands of daily living independently place him or her at risk.
         d. Socioeconomic and demographic factors. Lower socioeconomic status, being Caucasian, and being female are considered risk factors for long-term care.
         e. Marital status, living arrangement, and the informal support network. Living alone without resources for home care and few or no relatives living nearby to provide informal care are factors of high risk for institutionalization.
      2. Attitudinal factors
         a. Old persons in general are opposed to the use of institutions. Many view them as "places to go to die."
   C. Elder abuse
      1. It has been estimated that 10 percent of individuals over age 65 are the victims of abuse or neglect.
      2. The abuser is often a relative who lives with the elderly person and may be the assigned caregiver.
      3. Factors that contribute to abuse
         a. Longer life
         b. Dependency
         c. Stress
         d. Learned violence
      4. Identifying elder abuse
   D. Suicide

1. Persons over 65 years of age represent a disproportionately high percentage of individuals who commit suicide.
2. Twenty-five percent of all suicides are committed by this age group, and suicide is now a leading cause of death among the elderly.
3. The group at highest risk appears to be white men who are recently bereaved, living alone, experiencing anxiety due to financial instability, and have undertreated mood disorders.

VII. Application of the Nursing Process
  A. Assessment. Assessment of the elderly must consider the possible biological, psychological, sociocultural, and sexual changes that occur in the normal aging process.
    1. Age alone does not preclude that these changes have occurred, and each client must be assessed as a unique individual.
  B. Diagnosis/outcome identification
    1. Nursing diagnoses that relate to physiological changes in the aging individual may include any or all of the following:
      a. Risk for trauma.
      b. Hypothermia.
      c. Decreased cardiac output.
      d. Ineffective breathing pattern.
      e. Risk for aspiration.
      f. Impaired physical ability.
      g. Imbalanced nutrition, less than body requirements.
      h. Constipation.
      i. Stress incontinence.
      j. Urinary retention.
      k. Sensory-perceptual alteration.
      l. Sleep pattern disturbance.
      m. Pain.
      n. Self-care deficit.
      o. Risk for impaired skin integrity.
    2. Psychosocially related nursing diagnoses that may be a consideration include:
      a. Altered thought processes.
      b. Dysfunctional grieving.
      c. Risk for suicide.
      d. Powerlessness.
      e. Self-esteem disturbance.
      f. Fear.
      g. Body image disturbance.
      h. Altered sexuality patterns.
      i. Sexual dysfunction.
      j. Social isolation.
      k. Risk for trauma (elder abuse).
      l. Caregiver role strain.
    3. Outcome criteria are identified for measuring the effectiveness of nursing care.

C. Planning/implementation
1. Nursing care of the aging individual is aimed at protection from injury due to age-related physical changes or altered thought processes related to cerebral changes.
2. The nurse is also concerned with preservation of dignity and self-esteem in an individual who may have come to be dependent on others for his or her survival.
3. **Reminisence therapy** is encouraged.
4. Assistance is provided with self-care deficits while encouraging independence to the best of his or her ability.
D. Evaluation is based on accomplishment of previously established outcome criteria.

VIII. Summary
IX. Critical Thinking Exercise
X. Review Questions

ANSWERS TO CRITICAL THINKING EXERCISES

1. Dysfunctional grieving related to loss of husband/home/independence

2. a. Mrs. M. will begin progression through grief process by discussing her feelings about her losses.
   b. Mrs. M. will eat sufficient food to begin gaining weight.

3. Her loss of independence

CASE STUDY FOR USE WITH STUDENT LEARNING

Read the following case study and answer the questions that follow.

Seventy-seven-year-old Angie had been a widow for 20 years. She was fiercely independent, and had run her small farm with minimal assistance since her husband died. In the last few years, her children had noticed that Angie had become increasingly forgetful. First she began forgetting the birthdays of her children and grandchildren, which was highly unlike her. Recently, she forgot that she was supposed to visit her son and his family, and failed to show up at the designated time. Last week when her daughter visited, she found a tea kettle on the stove that had burned dry when Angie forgot she had started it. Yesterday, her daughter received a call from Angie's nearest neighbor who found Angie wandering around in his field unprotected from the cold. At Angie's children's request the family physician admits Angie to the hospital, where she is placed on the geropsychiatric unit.

1. Identify relevant assessment data from the information given.

2. What are the two priority nursing diagnoses for Angie?

3. Describe some nursing interventions for assisting Angie with the two nursing diagnoses identified.

4. Describe relevant outcome criteria for evaluating nursing care for Angie.

TEST QUESTIONS

Situation: As Eleanor, age 79, became increasingly unable to fulfill her self-care needs, her children, who lived in a distant city, agreed it would be best for her to move to a nursing home near them. The following questions pertain to Eleanor.

1. Eleanor became depressed when she knew she would have to sell her home that she had lived in for more than 50 years. The physician prescribed an antidepressant for Eleanor. Which of the following physiological changes in the elderly may require special consideration when prescribing psychotropic medications for them?
   - a. Changes in cortical and intellectual functioning
   - b. Changes in cardiac and respiratory functioning
   - • c. Changes in liver and kidney functioning
   - d. Changes in endocrine and immune functioning

2. Eleanor does not respond to the antidepressant medication and becomes more depressed. She tells the nurse, "I don't want to live here. I would rather die than live here." After hearing Eleanor make this statement, the nurse would be expected to add which of the following nursing diagnoses to Eleanor's care plan?
   - a. Risk for self-mutilation
   - • b. Risk for suicide
   - c. Risk for violence toward others
   - d. Risk for injury

3. When Eleanor does not respond to the antidepressant medication, the physician considers another therapy. Which of the following is he likely to choose?
   - • a. Electroconvulsive therapy
   - b. Neuroleptic therapy
   - c. An antiparkinsonian agent
   - d. Anxiolytic therapy

4. Eleanor begins to show improvement, and the physician orders additional therapy for her. Which of the following therapies is most likely to help alleviate depression in Eleanor?
    a. Behavior therapy
    b. Group therapy
    c. Orientation therapy
    • d. Reminiscence therapy

5. Which of the following nursing interventions would help Eleanor be as independent as possible in her self-care activities?
    a. Assign a variety of caregivers so that one person doesn't become used to doing everything for Eleanor.
    b. Allow Eleanor a specified amount of time to complete ADLs, then finish them for her.
    c. Tell her at the beginning of each day what is expected of her that day.
    • d. Allow her pattern of ADLs to follow her home routine as closely as possible.

6. The most common type of psychopathology in the elderly is:
    • a. Dementing disorders.
    b. Hypochondriasis.
    c. Anxiety disorders.
    d. Personality disorders.

7. Studies have indicated that the most critical factor discriminating between the elderly who remain in the community and those who must be institutionalized is:
    a. A healthy self-esteem.
    b. Strong spirituality.
    • c. Interpersonal relationships.
    d. Absence of mental illness.

8. In what way is learning ability affected by increasing age?
    a. The ability to learn diminishes with age.
    • b. Elderly individuals require increased amount of time for learning.
    c. Intellectual functioning declines with age.
    d. Long-term memory deteriorates with age.

9. Which of the following manifestations of elder abuse could be classified as *neglect*?
    a. Unexplained venereal disease
    b. Sudden lack of sufficient funds for daily living expenses

c. Excessive anxiety
- d. Lack of necessary supervision

10. Which of the following statements is true regarding physical changes in the elderly individual?
    a. There is an increase in production of gastric acid in the stomach.
    b. Loss of muscle mass occurs more slowly in women than in men.
- c. A decreased level of thyroid hormones causes a lowered basal metabolic rate.
    d. Changes in the immune system lead to an increased inflammatory response that results in delayed healing.

CHAPTER 24. COMMUNITY MENTAL HEALTH NURSING

CHAPTER FOCUS

The focus of this chapter is on nursing care of psychiatric clients in the community setting, using the framework of the model of public health: primary, secondary, and tertiary prevention. Emphasis is given to the chronically mentally ill and the homeless mentally ill. Nursing care is presented in the context of the six steps of the nursing process.

LEARNING OBJECTIVES

After reading this chapter, the student will be able to:
1. Discuss the changing focus of care in the field of mental health.
2. Define the concepts of care associated with the public health model.
3. Discuss primary prevention of mental illness within the community.
4. Identify populations at risk for mental illness within the community.
5. Discuss nursing intervention in primary prevention of mental illness within the community.
6. Discuss secondary prevention of mental illness within the community.
7. Describe treatment alternatives related to secondary prevention within the community.
8. Discuss tertiary prevention of mental illness within the community as it relates to the chronically and homeless mentally ill.
9. Relate historical and epidemiological factors associated with caring for the chronically and homeless mentally ill within the community.
10. Identify treatment alternatives for care of the chronically and homeless mentally ill within the community.
11. Apply the nursing process to care of the chronically and homeless mentally ill within the community.

KEY TERMS

deinstitutionalization
prospective payment
case management
community
shelters
mobile outreach units

diagnostically related groups (DRGs)
primary prevention
secondary prevention
tertiary prevention
store-front clinics

CHAPTER OUTLINE/LECTURE NOTES

I.   The Changing Focus of Care

A. Before 1840, there was no known treatment for the mentally ill, who were removed from the **community** to a place where they could do no harm to themselves or others.

B. In 1841, Dorothea Dix, a former school teacher, started a campaign that resulted in the establishment of a number of hospitals for the mentally ill.

C. The mentally ill population grew faster than the number of hospitals did, creating overcrowding and poor conditions.

D. In the 1940s and 1950s, a number of constitutional acts were passed, attempting to improve the quality of care for the mentally ill.

E. In 1963, the Community Mental Health Centers Act was passed. It called for the construction of community health centers.

F. **Deinstitutionalization** (the closing of state mental hospitals and discharging of mentally ill individuals) had begun.

G. Federal funding was reduced, however, and the number of community health centers was diminished.

H. Cost containment by **prospective payment** was initiated in 1983, drastically affecting the amount of reimbursement for health care services.

I. Clients are being discharged from the hospital with a greater need for aftercare than in the past, when hospital stays were longer. Outpatient services have become an essential part of the mental health care system.

II. The Public Health Model

A. **Primary prevention**
   1. Primary prevention is defined as reducing the incidence of mental disorders within the population.
   2. Nursing in primary prevention is focused on targeting groups at risk and providing educational programs.

B. **Secondary prevention**
   1. Reducing the prevalence of psychiatric illness by shortening the course (duration) of the illness
   2. Accomplished through early identification of problems and prompt initiation of effective treatment

C. **Tertiary prevention**
   1. Reducing the residual defects that are associated with severe or chronic mental illness
   2. Accomplished by preventing complications of the illness and promoting achievement of each individual's maximum level of functioning

III. The Community as Client

A. Primary prevention
   1. To identify stressful life events that precipitate crises and target the relevant populations at risk
   2. To intervene with these high-risk populations to prevent or minimize harmful consequences
   3. Populations at risk
      a. Individuals experiencing maturational crises
         (1) Adolescence

      (2) Marriage

      (3) Parenthood

      (4) Midlife

      (5) Retirement

   b. Individuals experiencing situational crises

      (1) Poverty

      (2) High rate of life change events

      (3) Environmental conditions

      (4) Trauma

B. Secondary prevention

  1. Early detection and prompt intervention with individuals experiencing mental illness symptoms

  2. Populations at risk

   a. Individuals experiencing maturational crises

      (1) Adolescence

      (2) Marriage

      (3) Parenthood

      (4) Midlife

      (5) Retirement

   b. Individuals experiencing situational crises

      (1) Nursing care at the secondary level of prevention with clients undergoing situational crises occurs only if crisis intervention at the primary level failed and the individual is unable to function socially or occupationally.

C. Tertiary prevention

  1. The chronically mentally ill

   a. Historical and epidemiological aspects

      (1) From 1955 to 1992, inhabitants of public mental hospitals dropped from more than 500,000 to approximately 120,000.

      (2) Deinstitutionalization occurred so rapidly that there was not sufficient time for planning for the needs of these individuals before they reentered the community.

      (3) The Coalition of Psychiatric Nursing Organizations (COPNO) has outlined the following essential services for mental health reform to assist the chronically mentally ill:

      (a) Primary care mental health services.

      (b) Universal access to a basic mental health package.

      (c) Long-term care.

      (d) Managed care.

   b. Treatment alternatives

      (1) Community mental health centers

      (2) Day-evening treatment/partial hospitalization programs

      (3) Community residential facilities

      (4) Psychiatric home health care

        (a) Care for the caregivers

2. The homeless mentally ill
    a. Historical and epidemiological aspects
        (1) The number of homeless in the United States has been estimated at somewhere between 250,000 and 4 million.
    b. Who are the homeless?
        (1) Age
        (2) Gender
        (3) Families
        (4) Ethnicity
    c. Mental illness and homelessness
        (1) It is thought that approximately 20 to 25 percent of the single adult homeless population suffers from some form of severe and persistent mental illness.
    d. Types of mental illness among the homeless
        (1) Most common: schizophrenia
        (2) Bipolar affective disorder
        (3) Substance abuse and dependence
        (4) Depression
        (5) Personality disorders
        (6) Organic mental disorders
    e. Contributing factors to homelessness among the mentally ill
        (1) Deinstitutionalization
        (2) Poverty
        (3) A scarcity of affordable housing
        (4) Lack of affordable health care
        (5) Domestic violence
        (6) Addiction disorders
    f. Community resources for the homeless
        (1) Interfering factors
            (a) Residential instability
            (b) Seasonal mobility
            (c) Migration
        (2) Health issues
            (a) Alcoholism
            (b) Thermoregulation
            (c) Rising incidence of tuberculosis
            (d) Dietary deficiencies common
            (e) Sexually transmitted diseases
            (f) Special health needs of homeless children
        (3) Types of resources available
            (a) Homeless **shelters**
            (b) Health care centers and **store-front clinics**
            (c) **Mobile outreach units**
    g. The homeless client and the nursing process: a case study
        (1) Assessment

(2) Diagnosis/outcome identification

(3) Plan/implementation

(4) Evaluation

IV. Summary

V. Review Questions

LEARNING ACTIVITY

Concepts and Terms Associated with Community Mental Health Nursing

Fill in the blanks of the statements below with the following terms and concepts associated with community mental health nursing.

deinstitutionalization	case management
DRGs	mobile outreach units
primary prevention	day treatment programs
secondary prevention	community
tertiary prevention	homelessness

1. In _____, volunteers and paid professionals form teams to drive or walk around and seek out homeless persons who are in need of assistance.

2. Nurse Jones visits Sam, who has chronic schizophrenia, in his home to give him his monthly injection of antipsychotic medication. This is an example of _____.

3. The release of thousands of chronically mentally ill individuals from state hospitals into the community setting is called _____.

4. The concept defined in #3 has been identified as a contributing factor to _____ among the mentally ill.

5. The term _____ refers to a group of people living in close proximity and having some dependency on each other.

6. The American Nurses Association has endorsed _____ as an effective method of providing care for clients in the community who require long-term assistance.

7. _____ are designed to ease the transition from hospitalization to community living.

8. _____, directed at control of Medicare costs, have reduced the length of hospital stays for psychiatric clients and increased the importance of aftercare.

9. Teaching a class in prepared childbirth education is an example of _____.

10. Caring for a widow who has been hospitalized for major depression is an example of _____.

TEST QUESTIONS

Situation: Victor is a 47-year-old man with schizophrenia. He lives with his 67-year-old mother, who has always managed his affairs. He has never been employed. Recently his mother had to have an emergency cholecystectomy, at which time Victor suffered an exacerbation of his psychosis and was hospitalized.

1. Victor's hospitalization represents an example of which of the following?
    - a. Primary prevention
 - b. Secondary prevention
    - c. Tertiary prevention
    - d. None of the above

2. On discharge from the hospital, Victor's physician refers him for nursing case management. Which of the following statements *best* describes case management?
    - a. Reducing residual defects associated with chronic mental illness
    - b. Provision of cost-effective care based on need
 - c. Long-term coordination of needed services by multiple providers
    - d. Recognition of symptoms and provision of treatment

3. Victor's case manager makes arrangements for psychiatric home health care. Which of the following criteria must be validated before Victor can receive this type of care?
 - a. His homebound status
    - b. His diagnosis of schizophrenia
    - c. His need for professional administration of medication
    - d. All of the above

4. Once a month, the home health nurse administers Victor's injection of haloperidol · (Haldol) decanoate. This nursing intervention is an example of:
    - a. Primary prevention.
    - b. Secondary prevention.
 - c. Tertiary prevention.
    - d. None of the above.

5. One of the major problems in attempting to provide health care services to the homeless is:
    - a. Most of them don't want help.
    - b. They are suspicious of anyone who offers help.
    - c. Most are proud and will refuse charity.
 - d. They have a penchant for mobility.

6. A recent increase in which of the following diseases has been noted among the homeless?
   - a. Meningitis
   - • b. Tuberculosis
   - c. Encephalopathy
   - d. Mononucleosis

7. Which of the following also are ongoing problems for many homeless individuals?
   - a. Alcoholism and thermoregulation
   - b. Sexually transmitted diseases, including HIV disease
   - c. Conditions related to dietary deficiencies
   - • d. All of the above

8. Which of the following interventions would be considered primary prevention for a homeless individual who lives at a shelter?
   - • a. Job training
   - b. A place to eat and sleep
   - c. Clean clothing
   - d. Nursing care

APPENDIX A
ANSWERS TO LEARNING ACTIVITIES

CHAPTER I. Mental Health and Mental Illness

Exercise I. Ego Defense Mechanisms

1. displacement
2. undoing
3. isolation
4. denial
5. introjection
6. identification
7. regression
8. compensation
9. repression
10. projection
11. suppression
12. Rationalization

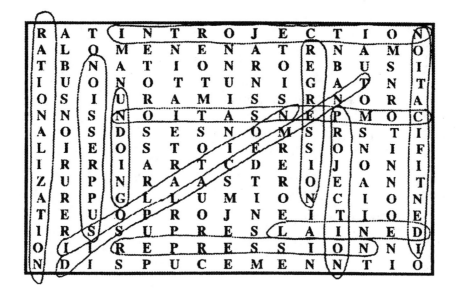

Exercise II. The Grief Response

1. Anger
2. Denial
3. Acceptance
4. Bargaining
5. Depression
6. Anger
7. Denial
8. Depression
9. Bargaining
10. Acceptance

CHAPTER 2. Concepts of Personality Development

Exercise I. Three Components of the Personality

1. id
2. superego
3. ego
4. id
5. id
6. ego
7. superego
8. id
9. ego
10. superego

Exercise II. Erikson's Stages of Development

1.	e	9.	i
2.	b	10.	f
3.	l	11.	j
4.	h	12.	a
5.	o	13.	p
6.	d	14.	k
7.	g	15.	c
8.	n	16.	m

CHAPTER 3: Biological Implications

Exercise I. Label the parts of the brain

<u> 1 </u> Frontal Lobe   <u> 4 </u> Medulla

<u> 5 </u> Parietal Lobe   <u> 7 </u> Cerebellum

<u> 2 </u> Temporal lobe   <u> 3 </u> Pons

<u> 6 </u> Occipital lobe

Exercise II. Crossword

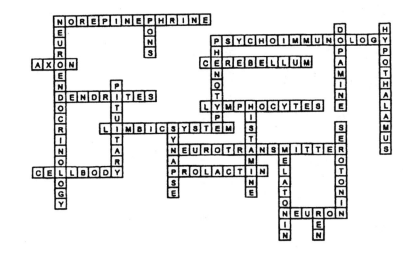

CHAPTER 4. Ethical and Legal Issues

Exercise I

1.	j	10.	i
2.	g	11.	k
3.	b	12.	c
4.	r	13.	o
5.	m	14.	n
6.	a	15.	h
7.	l	16.	f
8.	e	17.	q
9.	p	18.	d

CHAPTER 5. Relationship Development and Therapeutic Communication

Exercise I. Conditions Essential to Development of a Therapeutic Relationship
1. b
2. d
3. a
4. c
5. e

Exercise II. Phases of Relationship Development
1. b
2. a
3. c
4. b
5. d
6. a
7. c
8. d
9. d
10. c

Exercise III. Interpersonal Communication Techniques
1. Voicing doubt (T)
2. Belittling feelings (N)
3. Focusing (T)
4. Giving recognition (T)
5. Indicating an external source of power (N)
6. Reflecting (T)
7. Defending (N)
8. Exploring (T)
9. Verbalizing the implied (T)
10. Giving reassurance (N)
11. Restating (T)
12. Giving advice (N)
13. Giving broad openings (T)
14. Rejecting (N)
15. Requesting an explanation (N)

CHAPTER 6. The Nursing Process in Psychiatric/Mental Health Nursing

The Nursing Process: A Case Study

1. Assessment data
   a. Picks up a chair, as if to use it for protection. Threatened to harm anyone who came close to him in the department store.
   b. Talks and laughs to himself, and tilts his head to the side.
   c. Keeps to himself, and walks away when anyone approaches him.
   d. Appearance is unkempt. Clothes are dirty and wrinkled, hair is oily and uncombed, and there is an obvious body odor about him.

2. Nursing diagnoses
   a. Risk for other-directed violence
   b. Sensory-perceptual alteration (hallucinations)
   c. Social isolation
   d. Self-care deficit

3. Outcome criteria
   a. Sam has not harmed self or others.
   b. Sam is able to define and test reality.
   c. Sam approaches others in an appropriate manner for 1:1 interaction. Attends group activities voluntarily.
   d. Sam carries out personal care independently and willingly.

4. Some appropriate nursing interventions include:
   a. Remove dangerous objects from client's environment.
   b. Redirect violent behavior with physical outlets.
   c. Have sufficient staff available to indicate show of strength.
   d. Administer antipsychotic medication, as ordered (scheduled and p.r.n.).
   e. Encourage client to share content of hallucination.
   f. Help client to understand that even though the voices seem real to him, you do not hear the voices.
   g. Attend groups with client until he feels comfortable attending alone.
   h. Give positive feedback for voluntary interactions with others.
   i. Encourage client to be as independent with self-care activities as possible.
   j. Give positive feedback for self-care activities performed independently.

CHAPTER 7. Milieu—The Therapeutic Environment

Exercise I. The Interdisciplinary Team

1. Recreational therapist
2. Art therapist
3. Clinical psychologist
4. Chaplain
5. Dietitian
6. Music therapist
7. Clinical nurse specialist
8. Psychiatrist
9. Psychiatric staff nurse
10. Psychiatric social worker
11. Occupational therapist
12. Psychodramatist
13. Mental health technician

Exercise II. The Seven Basic Assumptions of a Therapeutic Community

1. e
2. a
3. g
4. f
5. b
6. d
7. c

CHAPTER 8. Intervention in Groups

Group Attendance

Students should prepare a written report of their attendance in a group describing:

a. Type of group attended.
b. Type of leadership identified.
c. Member roles identified.
d. Description of group dynamics.

CHAPTER 9. Intervening in Crises

Exercise I. Types of Crises

1. f
2. b
3. a
4. e
5. d
6. c

Exercise II. Crisis Intervention: Problem-Solving Process

1. Unresolved separation-individuation tasks:
    a. Unmet dependency needs
    b. Dysfunctional grieving

2. Realistic changes include:
    a. To develop a realistic and positive self-perception independent from parents.
    b. To relinquish need to secure personal identity through interaction with others.
    c. To progress through the grief process triggered by loss of previous lifestyle and come to terms with acceptance of the change.

3. Explore with Jane those aspects that cannot be changed. For example:
    a. Ted's job requires that he live in the new town.
    b. Jane's family will continue to live in the town from which they moved.

4. Alternatives include:
    a. Stay with Ted and accept the move (an alternative that is developmentally appropriate for Jane and that the nurse should encourage).
    b. Leave Ted and move back to hometown where relatives live (a decision based on developmental regression).

5. Jane will need to weigh the personal benefits and consequences of staying with Ted in the new town and working to accept the move or leaving him and moving back to live near her relatives.

6. Once Jane has made a decision, she may need assistance from the nurse to help her accept it and adapt to the change. Either decision will undoubtedly trigger a grief response, and assistance in progression to acceptance may be required. Jane must make the decision independently, based on knowledge and understanding of what each would mean for her. A decision to remain with Ted will require work on Jane's part to separate adaptively from her

parents and form an independent identity (tasks that have gone unfulfilled by Jane). New coping strategies will have to be developed.

CHAPTER 10. Psychopharmacology

Learning Activity: Psychotropic Medication Quiz

1. Increase levels of norepinephrine and serotonin
2. Sudden lifts in mood (may indicate suicidal intention)
3. Depending upon the medication, from 1 to 4 weeks
4. Tricyclic = amitriptyline (Elavil)
   MAOI = phenelzine (Nardil)
   SSRI = fluoxetine (Prozac)
5. a. Dry mouth (offer sugarless candy, ice, frequent sips of water)
   b. Constipation (increase fluids and foods high in fiber)
   c. Sedation (request physician to order given at bedtime)
   d. Orthostatic hypotension (teach client to rise slowly from a sitting or lying position; take vital signs every shift)
   e. Lowers seizure threshold (closely observe client, especially those with history of seizures)
6. Hypertensive crisis; nurse should be on the alert for symptoms of severe occipital headache, palpitations, nausea and vomiting, nuchal rigidity, fever, sweating, marked increase in blood pressure, chest pain, coma. Client must avoid foods high in tyramine, such as aged cheeses, pickles herring preserved meats, beer, wine, chocolate, sour cream, yogurt, over-the-counter cold medications, diet pills.
7. Mania. Lithium has a lag time of 1 to 3 weeks. Antipsychotics are prescribed to decrease the hyperactivity on an immediate basis until the lithium can take effect.
8. Therapeutic range: 0.6 to 1.5 mEq/L. Initial signs and symptoms of lithium toxicity are blurred vision, ataxia, tinnitis, persistent nausea and vomiting, severe diarrhea.
9. a. Give with food.
   b. Ensure client gets adequate sodium in diet.
   c. Ensure client drinks 2500 to 3000 cc fluid per day.
   d. Check for lithium levels before administering dose.
   e. Monitor client's intake and output.
   f. May need to instruct client on diet to prevent weight gain.
10. CNS depression
11. Benzodiazepines: chlordiazepoxide (Librium) and diazepam (Valium)
12. Drowsiness, sedation, confusion, orthostatic hypotension
13. Client must be instructed not to stop taking the drugs abruptly.
14. Decreases levels or activity of dopamine
15. Chlorpromazine (Thorazine) and fluphenazine (Prolixin)
16. Decreased libido; retrograde ejaculation; gynecomastia; amenorrhea; weight gain
17. Sore throat, fever, and malaise
18. Severe muscle rigidity, fever up to 107°F, tachycardia, tachypnea, fluctuations in blood pressure, diaphoresis, and rapid deterioration of mental status to stupor and coma
19. a. Pseudoparkinsonism (tremor, shuffling gait, drooling, rigidity)
    b. Akinesia (muscular weakness)
    c. Akathisia (continuous restlessness and fidgeting)
    d. Dystonia (spasms of face, arms, legs, and neck)
    e. Oculogyric crisis (uncontrolled rolling back of the eyes)
    f. Sometimes tardive dyskinesia is considered as an extrapyramidal system (bizarre facial and tongue movements; stiff neck, and difficulty swallowing)
20. Antiparkinsonian agents: benztropine (Cogentin) and trihexyphenidyl (Artane)
21. Depression and suicidal ideation

CHAPTER 11. Complementary Therapies

LEARNING ACTIVITY

Food Group: Fats, Oils & Sweets
No. of Servings: Use sparingly

Food Group: Milk, Yogurt & Cheese
No. of Servings: 2–3

Food Group: Meat, Fish, Dry
  Beans, Eggs & Nuts
No. of Servings: 2–3

Food Group: Vegetable
No. of Servings: 3–5

Food Group: Fruit
No. of Servings: 2–4

Food Group: Bread, Cereal, Rice & Pasta
No. of Servings: 6–11

CHAPTER 12. Delirium, Dementia, and Amnestic Disorders

Learning Activity:	Delirium	Dementia	Amnestic Disorder
1.	x		
2.			x
3.		x	x
4.		x	
5.	x		
6.			x
7.	x		
8.		x	
9.			x
10.		x	
11.	x		
12.	x		
13.	x		
14.		x	
15.			x

CHAPTER 13. Substance-Related Disorders

Exercise: Symptoms Associated with Psychoactive Substances

Drugs	Symptoms of Use	Symptoms of Intoxication	Symptoms of Withdrawal

CNS Depressants
Examples:
  Anxiolytics
  Alcohol
  Sedatives
  Hypnotics
	Relaxation, loss of inhibitions, lack of concentration, drowsiness, slurred speech	Aggressiveness, disinhibition, impaired judgment, incoordination, unsteady gait, slurred speech, disorientation, confusion	Tremors, nausea/vomiting, insomnia, seizures, hallucinations, irritability

CNS Stimulants
Examples:
  Amphetamines
  Caffeine
  Cocaine
  Nicotine
	Hyperactivity, agitation, euphoria, insomnia, anorexia, increased pulse	Euphoria, grandiosity, fighting, elevated vital signs, nausea and vomiting, psychomotor agitation	Anxiety, depressed mood, insomnia or hypersomnia, craving for the drug, suicidal ideas (with amphetamines and cocaine)

Opioids
Examples:
  Opium
  Morphine
  Codeine
  Heroin
  Meperidine
	Euphoria, lethargy, drowsiness, lack of motivation	Euphoria, lethargy, somnolence, apathy, dysphoria, impaired judgment, slurred speech, constipation, decreased respiratory rate and blood pressure.	Craving for the drug, nausea/vomiting, muscle aches, lacrimation, rhinorrhea, piloerection or sweating, diarrhea, yawning, fever, insomnia

Hallucinogens
Examples:
  Mescaline
  LSD
  PCP
	Visual hallucinations, disorientation, confusion, paranoia, euphoria, anxiety, panic, increased pulse	Belligerence, impulsiveness, psychomotor agitation, increased heart rate and blood pressure, ataxia, seizures, panic reaction, delirium	The occurrence of a withdrawal syndrome with these substances has not been established.

Cannabinols
Examples:
  Marijuana
  Hashish
	Relaxation, talkativeness, lowered inhibitions, euphoria, mood swings	Impaired judgment, loss of recent memory, tremors, muscle rigidity, conjunctival redness, panic, paranoia	If high doses are used for a prolonged period, symptoms of nervousness, tremor, insomnia and restlessness may occur upon cessation of use.

Inhalants Examples: Gasoline, lighter fluid, varnish remover, rubber cement, cleaning fluid, spray paint, typewriter correction fluid	(Same as CNS depressants)	Belligerence, apathy, assaultiveness, impaired judgment, dizziness, nystagmus, slurred speech, unsteady gait, lethargy, depressed reflexes, tremor, blurred vision, stupor or coma, euphoria, irritation around eyes, throat, and nose	

CHAPTER 14. Schizophrenia and Other Psychotic Disorders

Exercise I. Behaviors Associated with Schizophrenia

1. g
2. d
3. o
4. n
5. m
6. a
7. h
8. k
9. b
10. i
11. c
12. j
13. e
14. l
15. f

Exercise II. Case Study
1. paranoia
2. delusion of grandeur
3. echolalia
4. imitation
5. nihilistic delusion
6. anhedonia
7. body rocking
8. regression
9. anergia
10. apathy
11. autism
12. delusion of reference

a. Altered thought processes
b. An antipsychotic medication
c. (refer to Chapter 10 for side effects of antipsychotic drugs)
d. Trust vs. Mistrust because of her extreme suspiciousness
e. Generativity vs. Self-absorption

CHAPTER 15. Mood Disorders

Learning Activity: Symptoms of Mood Disorders

1. c
2. f
3. a
4. d
5. b
6. b
7. e
8. a
9. e
10. a
11. b
12. e
13. f

CHAPTER 16. Anxiety Disorders

Learning Activity: Behaviors Associated with Anxiety Disorders

1. c
2. g
3. b
4. d
5. f
6. a
7. c
8. e
9. d
10. f
11. b
12. c
13. g
14. e
15. d

CHAPTER 17. Anxiety-Related Disorders

Exercise I. Behaviors Associated with Somatoform Disorders

1. b
2. e
3. d
4. a
5. c

Exercise II. Behaviors Associated with Dissociative Disorders

1. c
2. e
3. a
4. g
5. b
6. f
7. d

CHAPTER 18. Disorders of Human Sexuality

Values clarification.   Students provide their own answers.

CHAPTER 19. Eating Disorders

Learning Activity: Symptoms of Eating Disorders

	Anorexia Nervosa	Bulimia Nervosa	Obesity
1.	X	X	
2.	X		
3.			X
4.		X	
5.	X		
6.	X	X	
7.			X
8.	X		
9.		X	
10.			X
11.		X	
12.			X
13.	X	X	
14.	X	X	X
15.		X	

CHAPTER 20. Personality Disorders

Learning activity
1. d
2. j
3. f
4. a
5. e
6. i
7. c
8. h
9. g
10. k
11. b

CHAPTER 21. Children and Adolescents

Learning Activity: Disorders of Infancy, Childhood, or Adolescence

1. h
2. e
3. j
4. b
5. d
6. g
7. f
8. i
9. c
10. a

CHAPTER 22. Victims of Abuse or Neglect

Learning Activity: Behaviors of Abuse or Neglect

1. d
2. i
3. h
4. c
5. g
6. j
7. k
8. a
9. l
10. f
11. e
12. b

CHAPTER 23. The Aging Individual

Exercise: Case Study

1. 77 years old
   A widow for 20 years
   Lives alone on small farm
   Has always been very independent
   Has become forgetful in last few years
   Forgetfulness has become dangerous to self
   Starting to wander
   Has caring support system in son and daughter

2. a. Risk for trauma related to confusion, disorientation, and wandering
   b. Altered thought processes related to age-related changes that result in cerebral anoxia evidenced by memory loss, confusion, disorientation, and wandering.

3. See Table 23.3, "Care Plan for the Elderly Client," in the textbook.

4. The client:
   a. Has not experienced injury.
   b. Maintains reality orientation consistent with cognitive level of functioning.
   c. Can distinguish between reality- and nonreality-based thinking.

   Caregivers and client:
   a. Verbalize understanding of possible need for long-term care placement

CHAPTER 24. Community Mental Health Nursing

Learning Activity: Concepts and Terms Associated with Community Mental Health Nursing

1. mobile outreach unit
2. tertiary prevention
3. deinstitutionalization
4. homelessness
5. community
6. case management
7. day treatment programs
8. DRGs
9. primary prevention
10. secondary prevention